Elements
of Pharmaceutical Pricing

Elements
of Pharmaceutical Pricing

E. M. (Mick) Kolassa, Ph.D.

informa
healthcare

New York   London

Informa Healthcare USA, Inc.
52 Vanderbilt Avenue
New York, NY 10017

© 2008 by Informa Healthcare USA, Inc. (original copyright 1997 by The Haworth Press, Inc.)
Informa Healthcare is an Informa business (cover design by Thomas J. Mayshock, Jr.)

Library of Congress Cataloging-in-Publication Data

Elements of pharmaceutical pricing / E.M. (Mick) Kolassa.
    p. cm.
  Includes bibliographical references and index.
  ISBN-13: 978-0-7890-0333-1; ISBN-10: 0-7890-0333-3 (hard : alk. paper)
  ISBN-13: 978-0-7890-0334-8; ISBN-10: 0-7890-0334-1 (soft : alk. paper)
  1. Drugs--Prices--United States. 2. Prescription pricing--United States.
  3. Pharmaceutical industry--United States.
  I. Title.

HD9666.4.K65   1997
615'.'0688--dc21   97-10137

Visit the Informa Web site at
www.informa.com

and the Informa Healthcare Web site at
www.informahealthcare.com

Elements of Pharmaceutical Pricing

CONTENTS

ABOUT THE AUTHOR

E. M. (Mick) Kolassa, Ph.D., is a Vice President of the Strategic Pricing Group, Inc. of Marlborough (Boston) Massachusetts. Recognized as a leading authority in the field of health care goods and services pricing, he has also consulted extensively with companies in the packaged goods, sporting equipment, and entertainment industries. Dr. Kolassa has served as Director of Pricing and Economic Policy for Sandoz Pharmaceutical Corporation, where he instituted the company's first Pricing Department, as well as its Health Economics Department. He has also held pricing and marketing research positions with The Upjohn Company, Fidelity Mutual Savings Bank, and Old National Bank.

Dr. Kolassa has held academic appointments as Research Scientist and Assistant Professor of Marketing. His research focuses on the role of price in decision making and the management of the pricing function within organizations. He received his doctorate from the University of Mississippi.

Dr. Kolassa has written and lectured extensively on pricing strategies and on the management of the pricing function. He is the author of "Pharmaceutical Pricing at the Change of Millennia," published in the *Journal of Pharmaceutical Marketing & Management* (1996); "Creating a Pricing Department," published in *The Journal of Professional Pricing* (1995); and "Pricing Under Pressure," published in *Medical Marketing and Media* (1994). A frequent speaker at conferences in the United States and Europe, he serves on the Board of Advisors of the Pricing Institute and the Editorial Board of *The Journal of Pricing Strategy and Practice* and the *Journal of Pharmaceutical Marketing Practice.*

Preface

In the early 1980s, the standard approach to pharmaceutical pricing was to set the price of a new product higher than the market leader and enjoy the revenue. The few exceptions to this rule found no benefit to their lower prices and eventually raised them. These price increases were soon copied by other firms, who found the lack of price sensitivity provided an opportunity to spur sales growth with little effort–most firms quickly fell into a pattern of one or two large price increases annually.

Some major changes to the pricing environment sent a shock into the system. The Waxman-Hatch bill transformed generic drugs from a mere annoyance to a major market threat, and the emergence of managed care and hospital buying groups gave rise to new concerns about price sensitivity. Research and development departments in many firms focused much of their attention on creating agents that were similar in mechanism and structure to already marketed products, giving rise to the "me-too" era of new drugs.

The pharmaceutical industry reacted to these and other trends by following a new rule: price new products at or below the prices of competitors, hoping to eliminate price as an obstacle to product adoption (1). National account groups then set to work discounting from these already lower prices. The federal government further complicated the working environment by granting itself access to the best prices the pharmaceutical companies made available, effectively penalizing drug firms and their customers. These new laws also deprived the pharmaceutical firms of their most potent sales growth tool, price increases. The penalties for increases above the rate of inflation were high enough to convince most firms to rein in their increases.

[Haworth co-indexing entry note]: "Preface." Kolassa, E. M. (Mick). Co-published simultaneously in *Journal of Pharmaceutical Marketing Practice* (The Pharmaceutical Products Press, an imprint of The Haworth Press, Inc.) Vol. 1, No. 1 (#1), 1997, pp. xiii-xv; and: *Elements of Pharmaceutical Pricing* (E. M. (Mick) Kolassa) The Pharmaceutical Products Press, an imprint of The Haworth Press, Inc., 1997, pp. xi-xiii. Single or multiple copies of this article are available for a fee from The Haworth Document Delivery Service [1-800-342-9678, 9:00 a.m. - 5:00 p.m. (EST). E-mail address: getinfo@haworth.com].

Seeking order in this increasingly chaotic environment, many firms turned to mechanistic approaches to pricing. Hundreds of millions of dollars have been spent on pricing research studies to determine the perfect price point, and companies have relied on fairly simple, often misleading, survey research findings to build strategic plans. Rigid internal pricing protocols have been established (and often ignored) by many firms. This, together with the research just mentioned, provides many firms with an illusion of some control (2).

The net result has been continually lower launch prices that soon decay in an environment of price negotiations and the unfortunate situation that many within the pharmaceutical industry do not have faith that their products are priced appropriately (3). Failure to understand the role of prices in decision making has caused many firms to forego a significant amount of profit in the quest to remain competitive with other firms whose actions they often have not taken the time to explore and understand. Rather than taking place in an environment of collusion and price fixing, as alleged in the retail pharmacy class action suits, the pricing actions of most pharmaceutical firms in recent years have been reactive, haphazard, and driven by short-term considerations. Those actions have resulted in leaving a significant amount of money "on the table." Short-term thinking leads to uninformed, emotional decisions, which, I believe, describes the majority of pharmaceutical pricing decisions made in the past several years.

Many firms now acknowledge these facts and that their pricing has been less than satisfactory. My voice mail is filled with messages from recruiters ("head hunters") who have been retained to find highly skilled pricing professionals for pharmaceutical firms, but there are few, if any, who have the background these firms are seeking. The searches have become more desperate, and the salary offers rise to levels I could only dream of when I worked in that area.

It is my hope that this book will help create within these firms, and the industry, something that has been long overdue–the ability to "price on purpose," to make pricing decisions that are less emotional and more informed. This volume does not contain all the answers, but I believe it does pose many of the right questions to help those charged with pricing make informed decisions and understand the likely implications of their pricing actions before taking them. This information should lead to better, more profitable pricing in the industry. It is by this standard that I will judge the usefulness of this book.

REFERENCES

1. Kolassa EM, Banahan BF. Growing competition in the pharmaceutical industry: a response to the PRIME Institute report. Technical Report PPM 95-001. University, MS: Research Institute of Pharmaceutical Sciences, 1995.

2. Pharma pricing USA: a comprehensive review of pharmaceutical pricing in the mid-1990s. London: IMS Pharma Strategy Group, 1995.

3. Health economics in the USA: expectations, applications, & future directions. Plymouth Meeting, PA: IMS America Health Economics Solutions Group, 1996.

Pricing:
The Forgotten "P"

A . . . pricing is the moment of truth–all of marketing comes to
focus in the pricing decision. (1)

–Raymond Corey

INTRODUCTION

Most people involved in the field of pharmaceutical marketing
are aware of the "4 *P*'s" of marketing, also called the marketing
mix: product, promotion, place, and price. But most marketing
efforts, with rare exceptions, are focused on the product and promotion, with virtually no thought given to distribution issues (place)
and very little serious attention given to pricing. Nagle and Holden
observed that the first three elements of the marketing mix–product,
promotion, and distribution–represent the firm's attempt to create
value in the marketplace, while pricing is used to capture some of
that value in the form of profits (2). Failure to develop and execute
an appropriate pricing strategy usually results in the failure of the
firm to capture an appropriate share of the value of the product,
which translates into lower profits.

Working with several firms over the past few years, I have made
the same observation again and again: very few people in the pharmaceutical industry (or any industry, for that matter) pay close

[Haworth co-indexing entry note]: "Pricing: The Forgotten 'P'." Kolassa, E. M. (Mick). Co-pub-
lished simultaneously in *Journal of Pharmaceutical Marketing Practice* (The Pharmaceutical Products
Press, an imprint of The Haworth Press, Inc.) Vol. 1, No. 1 (#1), 1997, pp. 1-11; and: *Elements of
Pharmaceutical Pricing* (E. M. (Mick) Kolassa) The Pharmaceutical Products Press, an imprint of The
Haworth Press, Inc., 1997, pp. 1-11. Single or multiple copies of this article are available for a fee from
The Haworth Document Delivery Service [1-800-342-9678, 9:00 a.m. - 5:00 p.m. (EST). E-mail address:
getinfo@haworth.com].

attention to their prices. To be certain, account managers, contract managers, and others spend a great deal of time bringing prices down, but very few people are charged with assuring that the prices charged are appropriate and profitable.

As detailed in the following chapters, the field of pharmaceutical pricing is complex, convoluted, and often ambiguous, but it is not unfathomable. The failure to manage pricing within the industry is a symptom of a much larger problem, one that is shared by other industries: the rampant lack of knowledge about the market and the competition. It is astonishing how little product managers, marketing researchers, and their superiors know about the markets in which they compete. Failure to understand one's customers and one's competitors is certain to lead to poor pricing decisions. For many, failure to understand is compounded by the failure to learn and apply basic pricing principles in pharmaceutical markets.

THE NEW PRODUCT DILEMMA

New products are often greeted with enthusiasm in consumer markets, but new products in pharmaceutical markets are often seen as problematic. Despite the clinical value of the product, systems must be changed to accommodate the use of the new medication. Unfortunately, few companies work with their customers to ease the problem of new product inclusion, instead taking actions to force the adoption of the product into the system. This often results in a reaction by affected parties, who delay new product evaluation or take some other steps to forestall product uptake. Understanding the world in which the customer operates and taking steps to bring your new product into that world with the customer's workload in mind can enhance the adoption of new drugs.

MARKET SEGMENTS

Vital to appropriate pricing is an understanding of the various segments in which the company competes, especially the degree of price sensitivity within each segment. Legislation and litigation have forced companies to reconsider the segments they had previously identified, but few have done more than simply reclassify groups into new segments and establish arbitrary guidelines for discounting within each segment. There is also a considerable amount of confusion between the classification of segments and channel members, intermediaries that are vital for distribution or financing but do not play the role of customers in any traditional sense.

The tools and techniques discussed here have applications in each segment of the pharmaceutical marketplace. Many will find that too much attention has been paid to intermediaries in the distributive process that have wrongly been classified as market segments. Wholesalers and most retailers fall into this category and, except in the most rare of circumstances, these groups should not receive special price consideration.

The lack of market and competitive knowledge and the use of general assumption have seduced many in the industry to assign higher levels of importance and price sensitivity to several segments. Additionally, the typical approach to pharmaceutical marketing itself has fed this problem because those involved in the marketing of pharmaceuticals tend to focus on their products and to view every aspect of the market through the filter of their own impression of the products. This is the reason many promotional campaigns focus on the mechanism of action of a drug rather than its end benefit. These forces (product focus, lack of awareness of market and competitive issues, and a general lack of familiarity with pricing concepts) combine to bring about three "disorders" that must be corrected. These pharmaceutical pricing diseases are:

1. Fear of Pricing
2. Inverted Focus
3. Managed Care Myopia.

FEAR OF PRICING

This malady is manifested in two ways. First, because of recent legislation and litigation, many corporate attorneys (whose primary purpose appears to be sales prevention) have decided that the word "price" will not be uttered within the confines of the corporate campus and that any sources of pricing information may constitute an attempt to collude, thus forcing the firm to price in a vacuum of no information. This problem is compounded by the deeply held belief of many in the industry that the price of the product has taken on newfound importance and that any product, no matter how beneficial from a clinical perspective, will fail miserably unless it is priced at a discount. Thus deprived of market information on which to base pricing decisions, the company instead simply assumes that every new product must be priced low relative to the competition.

An examination of the pricing of recently launched products reveals that the fear of pricing is rampant. The first of the new products is Lescol®, by Sandoz (Table 1). Much has been written and said about Lescol, which may be the only successfully dis-

TABLE 1. New Product Launch Prices.

PRODUCT (launch) NRx Share Comparator		Price at Launch (AWP)	Price at Launch (ex-factory)	Difference @ AWP	Difference@ ex-factory
Lescol (4/94)	15.6%	$1.02	$0.85	−49%	−46%
Mevacor	29.7%	$1.98	$1.59		
Univasc (6/95)	0.4%	$0.50	$0.40	−50%	−50%
Vasotec	27.0%	$1.00	$0.80		
Prevacid (6/95)	3.4%	$3.25	$2.64	−10%	−13%
Prilosec	22.0%	$3.63	$3.03		
Zyrtec (1/96)	N/A	$1.71	$1.37	−11%	−15%
Claritin	53.0%	$1.93	$1.61		
Effexor (2/94)	4.9%	$2.00	$1.60	−4%	−8%
Prozac	27.8%	$2.09	$1.74		
Serzone (1/95)	3.2%	$1.66	$1.38	−23%	−23%
Prozac	27.8%	$2.16	$1.80		
Flonase (1/95)	15.6%	$38.88	$32.40	20%	20%
Vancenase AQ	28.8%	$32.40	$27.00		
Rhinocort (6/94)	8.1%	$27.00	$22.50	−13%	−13%
Vancenase AQ	28.8%	$31.01	$25.84		

counted product to hit the U.S. market thus far. As we will see, it cannot be argued that discount prices have been especially helpful to any of the other products under investigation that appeared to attempt this tactic. The Lescol discount of nearly 50% and its relative share (15% versus 30% for its major competitor, rendering a competitive index of 0.5 [.15/.3]) will be used for comparative purposes. Achieving a share equal to half that of its biggest competitor is a major accomplishment for the fourth product into a market, and Sandoz' combination of low price and intensive, high-spending promotion was essential in achieving this.

Univasc®, the Schwarz Pharma ACE inhibitor, was also launched at a 50% discount. This product, as the ninth ACE inhibitor brand to enter the market, would not be expected to capture a significant share, but even with its massive discount, Univasc has failed to achieve even one-half point of share. The ACE inhibitor market is a "loud" one, with a considerable amount of promotional noise. I believe that the lackluster performance of Univasc is testament to the observation that a product still requires a compelling clinical reason for being prescribed, and a low price won't make up for this shortcoming. A successful low price strategy requires a significant amount of promotional spending and a fair amount of luck. Univasc, apparently, has neither. Univasc's competitive index of 0.01 (one-fiftieth that of Lescol) is indicative of the need for more than simply a low price.

TAP's proton pump inhibitor, Prevacid®, was launched at a 10% discount to Prilosec®, Astra Merck's pioneer product which is on its way to becoming the biggest pharmaceutical brand in history. Many believed that a significant discount for Prevacid would be disastrous to the Astra Merck product. TAP, however, seems to have understood the costly mistake of deep discount pricing. It chose to price only slightly below Prilosec, allowing its representatives to claim that it is a little less costly, but not attempting to devalue the therapeutic class (and leave a lot of money on the table while doing so). Prevacid's competitive index of 0.15 is respectable, but not fantastic. It bears watching, however, as the product does have potential for some significant growth as physicians move from H_2 antagonists to PPIs.

Another product with potential is Pfizer's Zyrtec®, which competes with Schering's Claritin® in the nonsedating antihistamine market. Pfizer, too, chose a small discount (11%) versus the competition, essentially removing price as an obstacle to sales (a choice that will be addressed). Although the share data used for this analysis were collected too early to be of use in assessing Zyrtec's performance, many expect Zyrtec to capture a substantial share of the market, as much as half that of Claritin's. This success, again, comes from promotional might, not deep discounting.

Next we will consider two products that entered a very large competitive market: antidepressants. Wyeth-Ayerst's Effexor® and Bristol-Myers Squibb's Serzone® entered the market about a year apart but miles apart in terms of pricing strategy. Effexor was launched at essentially the same price as Prozac®, the biggest competitor, with a discount of less than 10%. Serzone, which was launched later, came to market priced 23% below Prozac. Although Effexor has earned a higher share of prescriptions than Serzone, its year-long head start makes for an unfair comparison between the two. One would expect, however, that if the market were price sensitive, Serzone should be enjoying a much higher share than it is. Serzone's competitive index of .115 compares with Effexor's index of .17. Effexor's sales are 50% higher than Serzone's, and its price is 20% higher, a combination that argues against the efficacy of price in moving products.

Another market with similar competitive entries is the inhalable steroids. Schering's Vancenase® leads that market with a share of nearly 29%. Astra launched Rhinocort® into this market in mid-1994 at a 13% discount and achieved a respectable 8% share for a competitive index of .275. Glaxo then launched Flonase® into this market at a substantial premium of 20% over Vancenase and has captured a 15.6% share in its first year, a competitive index of .54. The success of this product, with unit sales nearly twice those of Rhinocort's at a price about 40% higher, again argues against the use of price as a selling point.

Because we are not privy to the reasoning behind the pricing of the products that have been discussed here, it is difficult to evaluate the success of the approaches. From this sample, however, we see more high-priced successes than low-priced successes, and no high-priced failures. The role of price in the success of a pharmaceutical product may be more closely related to the firm's confidence in the product and its ability to market the product than to a physician's decision to prescribe it. Some firms, as stated earlier, apparently believe that a price slightly below the competition's will provide them with some advantage, or at least avoid a potential pricing problem.

The decision to price a new product 5% to 15% below the competition, and thus avoid pricing problems altogether, might be considered a lazy approach to pricing. Essentially, it is an admission that the competitor has already set a good price, and we will avoid problems by parking below it. It can also be construed as an admission that the new product is not quite as good as, or at least no better than, what is already on the market. If that is the truth, then it may not be a bad choice. But if the team selling the product believes it has any clinical advantages, the price chosen for the product argues against any such suggestion. The benefits of such a choice may be in peace of mind, but it must be admitted that, for most of these products, a 10% discount represents an opportunity cost of 10% of sales.

Deep discounting (in the 20%+ range) can be construed as either a bold move or an act of desperation. To my thinking, Sandoz exhibited boldness with a deep price differential and a big budget to sell the advantage of its low price. I am not prepared to grant the title of "bold" to others who have used deep discounts, as these prices appear to have been set in hopes that the prices would sell the products, and it didn't work. Those who understand pricing make informed decisions; those who fear pricing make mistakes.

INVERTED FOCUS

This problem has been aggravated by the fear of pricing, but many firms have long suffered from it. Inverted focus causes firms to price their products according to the firms' own biased assessment of the value of the products—or worse, according to costs. Additionally, because of their failure to understand their customers, these firms often introduce new products into the marketplace that are met with hostility as opposed to the open arms anticipated by the marketing team. This problem results in disappointing market performance and often is followed by rampant discounting in an attempt to "get the product moving."

As previously discussed, firms that understand their customers have a much better chance of competing successfully. Those who choose instead to focus their efforts internally, not taking the time or expending the effort to truly understand their markets, will continue to make costly and avoidable mistakes, as the next discussion outlines.

MANAGED CARE MYOPIA

In the late 1980s, many firms established account management groups to market (or, rather, sell to) managed care and other buyers perceived to be large and influential. These account managers then set out to define and describe managed care and its growing influence. Because selling to managed care was their job, they made sure the company took this emerging market very seriously, and they overstated the importance of managed care in product selection.

Convinced that managed care is only concerned about price, some firms found it virtually impossible to resist discounting to this segment, and account managers continually provided horror stories of closed formularies and "NDC lockouts" that required huge discounts to assure product use. Most firms in the U.S. have responded to these threats by offering generous discounts in exchange for favorable treatment and generally have not realized the gains they had expected.

Although it is true that managed care now accounts for more than 50% of the outpatient prescription market in the U.S., data from IMS indicate that few of the managed care plans have actually restricted the use of branded pharmaceuticals. In fact, there are indications that the growth of managed care is responsible for a significant proportion of the growth of sales for branded pharmaceutical products over the past few years and that the discounts provided to these payers have had little, if any, effect on product use.

Some managed care organizations, specifically the staff models such as Kaiser and Group Health, do have the ability to affect sales because they take possession of the products and dispense the prescriptions that are written by employee physicians. But this type of managed care organization (MCO) is declining in importance and losing "covered lives" to network, IPA, and PPO model systems, which contract with physicians rather than employ them. It has been estimated that the average physician in the U.S. participates in more than three such plans. This dilutes the influence of any one MCO. More important, the majority of these plans, including the pharmaceutical benefits managers (PBMs), do not have the ability to affect product use significantly. It is estimated that only 17% of outpatient prescriptions are paid for by plans that can have any effect on the sales of specific branded products. The rest either simply administer the reimbursement for prescriptions with no restrictions at all (8%) or offer incentives to dispense generics when off-patent drugs are prescribed (25%). This means that the bulk of the business for branded products is effectively free of constraints.

Most firms have been eager to contract with managed care organizations based on the threat of their ability to control use. Pharmaceutical marketers have bemoaned the shrinking of the unrestricted cash market, where patients pay for their own prescriptions, believing that this market offers greater opportunities for pricing flexibility and a higher rate of profit. This segment declined from over half the market just 2 years ago to approximately 38% in 1995. Yet this segment appears to be much more price sensitive than the managed care market, which uses generics at a lower level than the cash segment and offers costlier agents higher shares than the cash market. How can this be?

Two facts must be understood. First, when the patient must pay for the prescription, he or she must be sensitive to the cost, as the ability to pay will determine the likelihood of the purchase. The bulk of the cash segment is senior citizens on fixed incomes, and seniors tend to use more prescription drugs than younger patients. They request products with generic alternatives and lower cost agents. A patient covered by a prescription plan, like patients in most European nations, cares nothing about the cost of the medications. Physicians routinely ask patients whether they have prescription coverage, knowing that a prescription card means the patient will have the prescription filled, regardless of the cost.

But what about managed care? Won't it intervene? The head of pharmacy for a major plan that covers nearly 10 million people stated that the most common question asked in his operation is, "How do we deny payment for this claim?" This question is asked because the prescription for the "restricted" drug has already been dispensed. Retail pharmacists know that they can override most restrictions, fill the prescription, and receive reimbursement. The plans tend to focus their energies on reducing use of big-line items such as Zantac® and Prozac in their attempts to achieve savings. They simply can't control hundreds of thousands of physicians, 50,000 pharmacies, and millions of patients, not to mention the thousands of prescription products that achieve sales lower than the blockbusters. Over one-half of MCOs state that their efforts at cost control amount to nothing more than asking physicians to consider costs while prescribing.

Competition among managed care plans has grown intense, and the appearance of restrictiveness on the part of a plan, manifested by refusing to pay for prescriptions ordered by its doctor, results in dissatisfied members who will look for a less restrictive plan. Member satisfaction has become a key performance measure among managed care plans, and losing members while trying to restrict pharmaceuticals, which only account for approximately 10% of MCO spending, makes little sense.

Discounts to managed care organizations have been declining, mainly because of the costly requirements that equal discounts be given to the federal government, which accounts for approximately 15% of sales, and the price discrimination suit against manufacturers. Many companies have reined in their discounts to managed care in response to these external stimuli. But those who have reduced discounting have discovered that lower discounts bring higher net sales and have little impact on unit use.

THE NEED TO PRICE ON PURPOSE

The failure to take pricing seriously results in lower profit margins. It is that simple. Many firms appear to have surrendered pricing authority to their competitors or to their customers, neither of whom is at all concerned about the financial success of the firm. They may, in fact, benefit from the firm's demise. Companies must make serious commitments to invest in pricing skills and to use prices to capture the value of their products, not to lower their value. Profitable pricing requires constant attention and continual learning, and it requires an understanding within the firm that the role of price is to secure the financial well-being of the firm and *not* to move more unit volume.

This text is aimed at helping the firm develop and refine its pricing skills and move ahead profitably.

REFERENCES

1. Corey R. Industrial marketing: cases and concepts. 3rd ed. Englewood Cliffs, NJ: Prentice-Hall Inc., 1983.

2. Nagle TT, Holden RK. The strategy and tactics of pricing: a guide to profitable decision making. 2nd ed. Englewood Cliffs, NJ: Prentice-Hall Inc., 1994.

The Growing Importance
of Pharmaceutical Pricing

INTRODUCTION

While public officials in the United States often note the growth of health care spending, especially for pharmaceuticals, and point to this growth as an indication of the need for tighter controls on health care costs, few have acknowledged the inevitability of cost increases in a system that provides goods and services at little or no cost (1). It has been said that there is almost no limit to the amount of free medical care an individual is capable of using.

Even though many health care insurance plans are comprehensive packages of health care goods and services meant to provide an overall benefit, the components of the benefit are often budgeted and managed as separate entities, resulting in conflicts between budgetary authorities (2). Thus it has become common that the greater good of the total system is often subordinate to individual budget performance.

In February of 1993, a symposium on drug costs, organized by the American Society of Hospital Pharmacists, was conducted in Atlanta, Georgia. The proceedings of the symposium were published as a supplement to the *American Journal of Hospital Pharmacy*. Entitled "The Rising Cost of Pharmaceuticals: Understanding and Managing the Escalating Cost of Pharmaceuticals in Health Care Institutions," this supplement presented the views of hospital

[Haworth co-indexing entry note]: "The Growing Importance of Pharmaceutical Pricing." Kolassa, E. M. (Mick). Co-published simultaneously in *Journal of Pharmaceutical Marketing Practice* (The Pharmaceutical Products Press, an imprint of The Haworth Press, Inc.) Vol. 1, No. 1 (#1), 1997, pp. 13-20; and: *Elements of Pharmaceutical Pricing* (E. M. (Mick) Kolassa) The Pharmaceutical Products Press, an imprint of The Haworth Press, Inc., 1997, pp. 13-20. Single or multiple copies of this article are available for a fee from The Haworth Document Delivery Service [1-800-342-9678, 9:00 a.m. - 5:00 p.m. (EST). E-mail address: getinfo@haworth.com].

pharmacists, administrators, physicians, and ethicists on the topic of rising pharmaceutical costs (3). The intent of the symposium was to develop recommendations on the control of expenditures for medications. The final statement of the participants recommended that new pharmaceutical products be evaluated in a manner similar to that used to assess the value of capital expenditures. This evaluation would be the responsibility of the pharmacy department and the P&T (pharmacy and therapeutics) Committee. As with many such efforts in the past, there is little evidence that the past three years have seen any serious effort by hospitals or hospital pharmacists to develop such evaluation procedures.

Serious concern for the prices of new pharmaceutical agents is relatively recent. Herfindal noted that, prior to 1985, it was unusual for even a large hospital to add a new pharmaceutical product to its formulary that would have a budgetary impact greater than $10,000 per year (4). He noted that some drug inclusion decisions now involve budgetary impacts of well over $1 million annually.

Costly new pharmaceuticals could not have come at a less opportune time for most health care systems. Prior to the early 1980s, the majority of medical procedures and services were reimbursed on the basis of cost (5). Providers were compensated based on the cost of providing the service, plus a fee or markup. Under such a system, there was little, if any, incentive to control expenditures. In fact, the opposite occurred, as providers could increase their incomes by simply providing more services. Beginning in the late 1970s, however, programs were developed and regulations were drafted and implemented to hold down health care costs, and the concept of managed care began to take hold.

In 1982, the enactment of the Tax Equity and Fiscal Responsibility Act (TEFRA) changed the basis of hospital reimbursement for procedures and services provided to Medicare patients from a cost-based program in which hospitals and other providers of health care billed the Medicare system on the basis of the costs incurred in delivering care, plus a markup, to one in which a per-case payment limit was imposed, establishing a fixed amount of reimbursement for each covered procedure (6). This change in reimbursement basis, called "prospective payment," imposed a condition on hospitals that the institution must provide a service at or below the fixed rate reimbursement–without regard to the individual institution's costs or cost structure–or suffer an economic loss (5). Many managed care providers have also implemented such systems of reimbursement.

At approximately the same time as the imposition of the prospective payment system, the manufacturers of pharmaceuticals began to increase the prices of their existing products, in addition to bringing new medications to market at higher-than-traditional prices for pharmaceutical products (7, 8). These concurrent phenomena of rising drug prices and restrictions on a provider's or insurer's ability to recover costs resulted in the implementation of several approaches to control drug expenditures, the most widely used of which are the restrictive formulary and formal drug utilization review (DUR) programs.

By 1988, it was estimated that more than half of the hospitals in the United States were operating at a loss, with costs exceeding revenues (9). Weisbrod noted that prospective payment systems confront hospitals with incentives to be cost conscious and that the financial incentives are to cut costs, provided the quality of care does not suffer "too much" (10). He argues that prospective payment systems implicitly encourage health care providers to reduce the use of resources in areas that are costly and difficult to monitor. Citing such phenomena as the reuse of disposable filters for renal dialysis machines, Weisbrod suggests that such reductions would minimize revenue losses, but in ways that would not be socially efficient. The complexity of the evaluation and comparison of new or competing pharmaceuticals provides the opportunity to reduce costs while sacrificing quality without such sacrifice becoming obvious. Weisbrod terms such activities opportunistic behavior toward asymmetrically underinformed consumers.

THE FORMULARY

The most common mechanism for evaluating and controlling the use of pharmaceuticals within a health care system is the formulary, which is generally developed and managed by the Pharmacy and Therapeutics (P&T) Committee. The concept of a formulary was proposed as early as 1936 by the American College of Surgeons (ACS) (11). In its proposal, the ACS recommended the establishment of P&T Committees in hospitals for the purpose of preparing formularies or "drug lists." The acceptance of the P&T Committee and accompanying formularies is such that the Joint Commission on Accreditation of Hospitals (JCAH) has required the operation of a P&T Committee in each hospital since 1965.

According to Rucker and Schiff, the purposes of the formulary were to *promote rational prescribing* and to identify drugs of choice for specific indications (12). Early operation and evaluation of formularies focused on this key goal, with only incidental attention paid to the economic effects of formulary control.

Pellegrino, in 1965, argued that formularies and P&T Committees would "fail if they are used as a means to greater economy and efficiency or to 'regiment' the medical staff" (13). He asserted that the formulary is "essential to the improvement of patient care through critical attention to all aspects of hospital treatment." From these statements it is evident that the formulary system was being used, at least in some institutions, as a means of cost control as early as 1965. Contemporaneously, it was being argued before the United States Senate in 1967 that "the application of a carefully designed formulary theoretically provides the foundation for guiding clinicians in choosing the safest, most effective agents for treating medical problems" (12). This dichotomous view of formularies has been noted by Rucker as a problem in "*[k]eeping clear the distinctions between quality versus cost as the raison d'etre for formularies*" (emphasis added) (12). He observed that, because drug costs are borne by the hospital, P&T Committee members, including the directors of pharmacy, internalize objectives to reduce costs when attempting to accommodate the drug budget. According to Rucker, this leads to confusion about the primary purpose of the formulary.

OUTPATIENT FORMULARIES

Over the past decade, several studies have demonstrated that tight budgetary control of pharmaceuticals often results in increases in spending on other health care goods and services to offset any savings on drugs, a phenomenon known as the service substitution effect (14, 15). Other studies by Moore and Newman and Smith and Simmons have shown that the imposition of these controls through outpatient formularies in the Medicaid setting does not even guarantee reduced spending on pharmaceuticals (16, 17). While some other studies in this area were questioned for their assumptions or methodologies, few, if any, studies have been produced that establish the ability of a restrictive formulary alone to save money in an outpatient setting (18).

Several cost control schemes, such as monthly prescription limitations and cost sharing, have also been shown to be less than optimal in controlling costs, because, as Nelson, Reeder, and Dickson found, restrictions or cost sharing can result in problems of underutilization that can have a negative effect on health and result in cost increases (19). The imposition of a maximum number of prescriptions per beneficiary has been shown to have severe negative consequences, increasing total costs by increasing hospitalizations and nursing home admissions (20).

Moore and Newman assert that advocates of restrictive formularies subscribe to what Demsetz has described as the Nirvana approach as a guide to regulation and control (21). Under this approach, managers and regulators search for discrepancies between the ideal, or perfectly operating, system and the existing situation. Any discrepancies lead to the conclusion that the existing situation (in this case an open formulary accompanying increasing costs) is inefficient and constitutes a market failure. They assume that tight regulation is the solution to the problem, disregarding the potential inefficiencies or defects of the regulatory approach.

This approach to controlling costs has met with a serious challenge, in the form of the Managed Care Outcomes Project (MCOP) by Horn and colleagues (22). This study found that restrictive formularies and mandatory generic substitution were associated with higher costs (both total costs and pharmacy costs) and lower levels of patient outcomes. As may be expected, many in managed care whose livelihoods depend on formulary management are seeking to discredit the study. Time will tell if the forces of reason win out over entrenched bureaucracies, but the future appears to hold promise.

Pharmaceutical companies are placing a great deal of faith in the ability of pharmacoeconomic studies to overcome price resistance. As Horn's recent experience demonstrates, even unbiased and well-balanced studies that conflict with the views (and self-interest) of those in charge of budgets cannot single-handedly overcome this mentality, and firms that believe their own studies will be more influential than the MCOP study and others will be sorely disappointed. As long as individuals within the system are charged with controlling drug expenditures, this silo approach to budgeting will continue. The way to overcome this myopic approach to the control of pharmaceutical costs is to establish and promote the value of pharmaceuticals in relation to other health care resources. In this endeavor, many related obstacles must be overcome, including:

- The common practice of tying physician and/or pharmacist compensation to the level of expenditures in the pharmacy budget. If an individual's pay is determined by the level of spending, he or she will take steps to minimize the budget and maximize his or her own income.
- The silo approach used by many health care systems, private and public. These systems develop perverse incentives, rewarding choices that are detrimental to the system as a whole. Significant efforts must be made to change this approach by building public awareness of the adverse consequences of this approach, by enlisting the support of public officials and other public figures to change the system, and by working with senior managers within health care systems to manage budgets on a more comprehensive basis.
- The lack of appreciation for the value of pharmaceuticals. Although patients think little of spending several hundred dollars for physician office visits and diagnostic procedures, they (and others) recoil at the thought of a drug costing as much. This is due, in part, to the failure of the industry to promote the value of pharmaceuticals and to sell the end result (lack of disease) instead of the chemical itself.

As long as these obstacles exist, there will be misguided efforts to control the use of pharmaceuticals, and these efforts will reduce the profitability of pharmaceutical research. Those charged with recommending or setting the prices and pricing strategies of pharmaceutical products must understand and manage this environment or risk significant declines in profitability.

REFERENCES

1. Goodman JC, Dolan EG. Economics of public policy. St. Paul, MN: West Publishing Company, 1985.

2. Kozma CM, Reeder CE, Lingle EW. Expanding Medicaid drug formulary coverage: effects on utilization of related services. Med Care 1990;28:963-76.

3. Gouvenia WA, ed. The rising cost of pharmaceuticals: understanding and managing the escalating cost of pharmaceuticals in health care institutions. Am J Hosp Pharm 1993;50(Suppl 4):S1-18.

4. Herfindal ET. Formulary management of biotechnological drugs. Am J Hosp Pharm 1989;46:2516-20.

5. Choich R. Product and service compensation. In: Brown TR. The handbook of institutional pharmacy practice. 3rd ed. Bethesda, MD: American Society of Hospital Pharmacists, 1992.

6. Curtiss FR. Current concepts in hospital reimbursement. Am J Hosp Pharm 1983;40:586-91.

7. Smythe SM. Prescription pricing: a GAO evaluation. J Res Pharm Econ 1991;3(1):55-64.

8. Pryor D. Commentary: a prescription for high drug prices. Health Aff 1990;9:101-9.

9. Rosenstein AH. Health economics and resource management: a model for hospital efficiency. Hosp Health Serv Admin 1991;36:313-30.

10. Weisbrod BA. The health care quadrilema: an essay on technological change, insurance, quality of care, and cost containment. J Econ Lit 1991;23:523-52.

11. Danials CE, Wertheimer AI. Analysis of hospital formulary effects on cost control. Top Hosp Pharm Manage 1982;(Aug):32-47.

12. Rucker TD, Schiff G. Drug formularies: myths-in-formation. Med Care 1990;28:928-39.

13. Pellegrino ED. A physician appraises the formulary system. Hospitals 1965;39:77-80.

14. Bloom BS, Jacobs J. Cost effects of restricting cost-effective therapy. Med Care 1985;23:872-80.

15. Hefner DL. Cost effectiveness of a restrictive drug formulary. Washington, DC: National Pharmaceutical Council, 1980.

16. Moore WJ, Newman RJ. U.S. Medicaid drug formularies: do they work? PharmacoEconomics 1992;1(Suppl 1):28-31.

17. Smith MC, Simmons S. A study of the effects of formulary limitations in Medicaid programs. Admin Policy J 1982;2(2):169-98.

18. Rucker TD, Morse ML. The Medicaid drug program in Louisiana: critique of the Hefner-Pracon study. Am J Hosp Pharm 1980;37:1350-3.

19. Nelson AA, Reeder CE, Dickson WM. The effect of a Medicaid drug copayment program on the utilization of prescription services. Med Care 1984;22:724-36.

20. Soumerai SB, Avorn J, Ross-Degnan D, Gortmaker S. Payment restrictions for prescription drugs under Medicaid: effects on therapy, cost, and equity. N Engl J Med 1987;317:550-6.

21. Demsetz H. Information and efficiency: another viewpoint. J Law Econ 1966;22:1-22.

22. Horn SD, Sharkey PD, Tracy DM, Horn CE, James B, Goodwin F. Intended and unintended consequences of HMO cost-containment strategies: results from the Managed Care Outcomes Project. Am J Managed Care 1996;2:253-64.

Prices, Politics, and Problems– A Pricing Philosophy

INTRODUCTION

The prices charged for pharmaceuticals have been the subject of public policy scrutiny for decades. Politicians wishing to demonstrate their concern for the welfare of citizens have periodically determined that the prices charged for medications provide a relatively risk-free platform to show that concern. The pharmaceutical industry, in turn, goes into a defensive posture and pleads the need for research as its only defense for prices. The net result, inevitably, is that the industry loses ground, either through a damaged public image or through the loss of some pricing freedom.

Although research is the heart of the branded pharmaceutical industry, the public has not shown willingness to accept that as an argument for "high prices." The problem lies in the failure of the industry to establish–and hence the public's failure to understand– the value of pharmaceuticals relative to other health care goods and services. Until that relationship is established and communicated in a credible and understandable manner, pharmaceutical firms will have continuous problems with their prices and public policy.

Rather than listing exhaustively the litany of reasons for the poor reception of pharmaceutical prices or the elements that make the pharmaceutical industry such a wonderful target for critics, let us consider the general aspects of the problem and seek solutions. To

[Haworth co-indexing entry note]: "Prices, Politics, and Problems–A Pricing Philosophy." Kolassa, E. M. (Mick). Co-published simultaneously in *Journal of Pharmaceutical Marketing Practice* (The Pharmaceutical Products Press, an imprint of The Haworth Press, Inc.) Vol. 1, No. 1 (#1), 1997, pp. 21-27; and: *Elements of Pharmaceutical Pricing* (E. M. (Mick) Kolassa) The Pharmaceutical Products Press, an imprint of The Haworth Press, Inc., 1997, pp. 21-27. Single or multiple copies of this article are available for a fee from The Haworth Document Delivery Service [1-800-342-9678, 9:00 a.m. - 5:00 p.m. (EST). E-mail address: getinfo@haworth.com].

begin, pharmaceuticals are "negative goods." As products used to correct an already existing problem, they are intended to lessen the negative effects of a condition as opposed to adding positive effects. Gasoline is a classic "negative good." We don't purchase it because we want to; we do so because we must. Like medications, gasoline is considered a necessity for a normal life, but it is not positively desired. More important, although the individual consumer can decide when to buy gasoline and can make decisions about the purchase, the consumer has little control over medication purchases, which tend to be directed purchases. For this reason, pharmaceuticals will always be viewed negatively.

What can companies do to at least moderate the criticism? As already mentioned, pleading the need to generate research funding is not the answer. Perhaps, as with the case of gasoline and other "negative goods," the answer lies in communicating some positive aspects of the products while acknowledging that a sizable proportion of the market will never admit to the value of the products. Premium-grade gasolines are positioned to enhance the performance of a car and to protect an investment, and pharmaceuticals can be positioned similarly.

A PHARMACEUTICAL PRICING PHILOSOPHY

The unique nature of pharmaceuticals, being the product of profit-seeking corporations but considered by many to be a "public good," has resulted in major differences between pharmaceutical markets and the so-called free markets. The fact that most pharmaceutical purchases are directed purchases and the fact that few patients can correctly be considered well-informed consumers are just two of the reasons pharmaceutical markets are unlikely to be truly free markets.

This is not to say that the development and marketing of pharmaceuticals will not continue to be a profitable—and noble—endeavor; it simply means that many of the tools and techniques for pricing and market analysis developed for free consumer markets will not have direct applicability in the market for medications. The discussion of pharmaceutical pricing research, which is presented in the section on the role of price in the decision to purchase, prescribe, or use pharmaceuticals, considers this from a market perspective, but we must reach an understanding on some key issues before that discussion.

Willingness to Pay

Pharmaceutical companies should rightly expect to be rewarded for providing value to the health care marketplace. Even most critics will agree with this statement. The problem arises when the industry's rewards and the value provided appear to be out of balance. This is more a problem of poor communication of value than of overpricing, but the latter is the impression held by many.

Economists specializing in public policy have developed a set of tests to determine the value of a program. These tests are based on the amount taxpayers or consumers state they would be willing to pay for a particular benefit from the program. For example, to measure the value of improved air quality in an area, researchers would ask residents to estimate the amount residents would be willing to pay to achieve cleaner air. The responses would then be averaged to compute the value consumers place on air quality and to evaluate the fairness and acceptability of a tax levy to bring about this quality.

These tests have been transferred into the realm of health care and are widely used in pharmacoeconomic studies in Europe. They have also been used in the United States, both for pharmacoeconomics and for pharmaceutical pricing research. Although the concept of willingness to pay is compelling, we must admit that, because of the distortions in our health care system due to differences in payment sources for health care and the lack of direct decision-making authority for patients, such measures may not only be impractical but also misleading.

Take, for example, the case of a treatment for Alzheimer's disease. The individual caring for the patient (the caregiver) could be asked, "What would you be willing to pay for this medication that stops the progress of the disease?" A typical response may be, "I would pay anything to help my wife (husband, mother, or father)." When pressed for a dollar amount, the respondent may give unrealistic figures because he cannot make a fully informed assessment of the value of the medication and may simply be grasping at straws in desperation. Such desperate measures are not uncommon in terminal, debilitating diseases and, in my opinion, the results of such lines of questioning provide little information of value in setting an appropriate price.

Your Money or Your Life

In health care markets, we are granted the unique authority, by virtue of the products that are developed, to charge whatever we wish. Because pharmaceuticals are a directed purchase, often reimbursed by a third party (but nearly as often not reimbursed), we have the peculiar ability to say to a patient "It's your money or your life." The prices charged for medications can, in fact, become a barrier that will deny some patients access to them, and we must keep this in mind, balancing company needs with patient needs and abilities when establishing prices and programs to assure as near universal access as is practicable.

UNDERSTANDING THE SITUATION

Polypharmacy

There are several medications on the market for which patients and payers willingly (apparently) pay several dollars per day. But the prospect of polypharmacy for many patients and the fact that the additive effect of several products at such prices can be prohibitive should give us pause before we attempt to charge similar prices for every product that is developed. Parkinson's disease provides a very good example of this situation.

It is not uncommon that a Parkinson's patient, who is likely to be retired and a Medicare beneficiary and the least likely to be covered by a prescription plan, takes two or more medications for Parkinson's: a dopamine product costing $2 to $3 per day, and a dopamine agonist or other agent costing from $3 to $5 per day. In addition, these patients often require antidepressants ($2 per day), antiarthritics ($2 per day), and perhaps medications for hypertension and/or high cholesterol, which add another $1.50 to $3 per day. It is not exceptional for the Parkinson's patient to spend between $10 and $20 per day for medication.

Although each of these medications may be priced appropriately by itself, when the additive effect of polypharmacy is considered, do the patients really receive this value? Must every new drug for Parkinson's cost $3 per day, especially if it will be used as an adjunct to current therapy and not as a replacement? Replacing a $3 drug with another $3 drug has no net financial impact on the patient, while adding a new $3 drug to a regimen that already costs $15 per day may force the patient into choices that benefit no one–foregoing one medication to afford another and compromising health or the increasingly common occurrence of self-imposed rationing, where the patient skips every other dose of needed medications to afford those medications. The prevalence of this phenomenon is unknown, but it should be measured and evaluated before the prices of new drugs in this and other therapeutic areas are set.

Reimbursement Status

Differences in reimbursement status dramatically alter the levels of price sensitivity and the economic effects of a product. For seniors, lack of Medicare coverage for outpatient prescriptions means that receiving injectable medicines in a physician's office, which is covered, is far less costly than oral agents. This and other examples point to the logical flaws in the system, flaws that must be considered.

A new drug that replaces a surgical or other mechanical procedure may offer significant savings, but the cost of the drug is borne by the pharmacy budget while the cost of the procedure is borne by the medical budget. Replacing evulsion or debridement–common procedures for nail fungus, decubitus ulcers, and other topical maladies–with a new medication brings about two major issues: shifting the cost of the disease to another budget area and shifting the financial reward of treatment from one entity to another.

During the Watergate scandal of the early 1970s, Deep Throat, the anonymous inside informant, told reporters to "follow the money." That advice should also be taken by those establishing prices for new pharmaceutical products. The shifting of financial responsibility from the medical to the pharmacy budget means the pharmacy will see an increase in its costs, perhaps without credit for savings elsewhere. Moreover, the physician who must prescribe the new agent may find that his or her income is dramatically reduced when the new drug is used because the procedures replaced by the drug have been a major source of income. In such circumstances it is foolhardy to assume that the savings provided by your new drug will be welcomed by the system.

Mandatory Discounts

Federal legislation introduced over the past few years has dramatically increased the complexity of pricing decisions. Discounts to favored customers must be evaluated in light of mandatory rebates to the Medicaid system and to other federal government entities. The ongoing discriminatory pricing litigation in federal courts will also alter the pricing landscape. Any pricing decision must now be made in light of these forces.

The Law of Unanticipated Consequences

The Omnibus Budget Reconciliation Act of 1990 (OBRA 90) effectively penalized companies for providing discounts. The government's attempt to share in those discounts had the effect of changing the economics of discounting, reducing the value of many customers when Medicaid rebates were calculated. The net result was the significant reduction of discounting activities in the pharmaceutical market, which reduced the revenue expected to be generated by the rebates (1). Just as the federal government's expectations were thwarted by the industry's response to the imposition of mandatory rebates, so, too, are marketing plans often foiled by the unanticipated consequences of pricing actions.

The market's failure to embrace the low-price strategies of Adalat CC®, Lotensin®, Plendil®, Univasc®, and a number of other agents launched in the past five years results from the failure of marketers—who were operating under the assumption that price sensitivity had risen in importance in the market—to understand the forces affecting product decisions. Similarly, the backlash over the restricted distribution of Clozaril® that resulted in the unbundling of the monitoring system the company put in place to protect patients was not due to any faults in the design of the program, but to a disregard of the potential backlash from pharmacists, who were excluded from the distribution process.

PRICING ON PURPOSE

Many of the problems encountered in the domain of pharmaceutical pricing have occurred because those involved in the decision were not proficient in the field of pharmaceutical pricing and because erroneous, but often logical, assumptions were made concerning the role and effects of price in the market. Pricing mistakes emerge from failure to consider all the potential consequences of pricing actions–failing to "price on purpose."

Pricing on purpose means that each price considered has been evaluated for its effect on the health care system and members of that system and balanced with a realistic assessment of the willingness and ability of those members to take action. As the cost of pricing mistakes increases, the need to price on purpose grows.

REFERENCE

1. Medicaid: changes in best price for outpatient drugs purchased by HMOs and hospitals. Fact Sheet, 08/05/94. GAO/HEHES-94-194FS.

Pricing Flow and Terminology

INTRODUCTION

How many of the following questions can you answer?

- Why is it that your new antihypertensive agent, which you priced 20% below your best-selling competitor, is perceived as being too expensive because it costs patients 20% *more* than your competitor?
- Do wholesalers really mark your products up by 20%, as implied by the AWP?
- Why is it that a generic priced 75% below your product is being advertised as offering "savings up to 40%"?
- How can prime vendor wholesalers make money on a contract that only allows a 2% markup?

If you cannot answer many, or any, of these questions, you are not alone. They are not difficult to answer. The problem lies in the fact that few people have *asked* them. Try them again after reading this chapter.

This discussion introduces the various terms and buzzwords of pharmaceutical pricing and addresses the different pharmaceutical prices that exist in the market. Although the term pharmaceutical market has often been used, there are, in fact, several pharmaceutical markets, each with its own set of prices and pricing methods. There are retail, hospital, and managed care markets; branded and

[Haworth co-indexing entry note]: "Pricing Flow and Terminology." Kolassa, E. M. (Mick). Co-published simultaneously in *Journal of Pharmaceutical Marketing Practice* (The Pharmaceutical Products Press, an imprint of The Haworth Press, Inc.) Vol. 1, No. 1 (#1), 1997, pp. 29-44; and: *Elements of Pharmaceutical Pricing* (E. M. (Mick) Kolassa) The Pharmaceutical Products Press, an imprint of The Haworth Press, Inc., 1997, pp. 29-44. Single or multiple copies of this article are available for a fee from The Haworth Document Delivery Service [1-800-342-9678, 9:00 a.m. - 5:00 p.m. (EST). E-mail address: getinfo@haworth.com].

generic markets; and chronic and acute markets. Each is approached somewhat differently.

It is important to define the common terms used in pharmaceutical pricing before we examine these various markets.

IMPORTANT TERMS IN PHARMACEUTICAL PRICING

As with all specialized areas, pharmaceutical pricing has its own vocabulary, complete with acronyms. Here is a list of common pharmaceutical pricing terms and their definitions.

Actual Acquisition Cost (AAC). Retail pharmacy reimbursement arrangements are often based on the AWP (see below) plus a fee. Knowing that retailers no longer pay the published AWP for prescription drugs, many payers attempted to reduce the reimbursement by discounting the AWP by 5% to as much as 20%. Because this system penalizes the pharmacies that are unable to secure significant discounts from wholesalers, some payers have instituted a payment schedule on the basis of actual acquisition cost plus a fee. Billing complexities and schemes, however, make it difficult to ascertain the actual acquisition cost.

Average Manufacturer's Price (AMP). This term was developed by the drafters of OBRA 90 and is used to describe the average price received by a manufacturer, after discounts, for products sold to the retail class of trade. The AMP is used for computing the rebates that are paid to state Medicaid programs.

Average Wholesale Price (AWP). Neither an average price nor a price charged by wholesalers, this figure is a vestige of earlier times. Few, if any, wholesalers even consider AWP today when pricing their prescription products. It is, however, commonly used by retailers and others who dispense medications as the basis for many pricing decisions. Due to its availability from many sources, the AWP is often used as a surrogate for actual prices when studying prescription price trends.

Cash Discount. Most pharmaceutical firms offer incentives to their customers for rapid payment of invoices. The most common terms offered are a 2% discount if the full bill is paid within 10 days of receiving the invoice. Thus a wholesaler that pays the regular ex-factory price actually pays only 98% of that price if it pays within 10 days. The wholesaler that sells at cost plus 3%, then, is actually charging a markup of roughly 5%.

Chargeback. This is the difference between the price a wholesaler pays a manufacturer (see WAC) and a lower contract price that has been negotiated by a hospital or managed care organization. Because of complexities of tracking products and some legal limitations, the chargeback system was developed as a means for discounted products to be sold through wholesalers. The wholesaler purchases the product at the normal list price and sells the product to hospitals or other contract customers at the discount price. The difference is then paid as a rebate to the wholesaler by the manufacturer. This rebate is called the chargeback.

Class of Trade. Under federal law, all businesses that sell to the same customer type must be eligible to receive equal pricing consideration, such as discounts and special offers. To assure compliance with this law, most pharmaceutical companies have developed lists of similar customers and grouped them into different classes of trade. Pricing schedules and tactics are then developed for each class of trade.

Direct Price. The price paid by retailers, before discounts, for products from those manufacturers who sell directly to nonwholesale accounts such as retailers, hospitals, private practice physicians, and public health clinics is called the direct price.

Earned Margin. Earned margin is a term used by some retail pharmacists to describe the difference between the AWP and the actual product cost, as paid to the wholesaler or manufacturer.

Ex-Factory Price. This is the actual selling price, before discounts, charged by the manufacturer (see WAC).

Gross Profit (Margin). The difference between acquisition or production cost of a product and its selling price is known as the gross profit margin. The gross profit margin does not include other costs of doing business.

Loss Leader. A loss leader is a retail promotional pricing tactic in which the retailer charges a price that is below cost to entice customers into the store, hoping that the customers will make additional purchases while there. In retail pharmacy, a loss leader is not always priced below actual cost, but below AWP. It can, however, be argued that the transaction is indeed a loss when factoring in the professional time and services required to fill a prescription. Still, a pharmacy loss leader does not imply selling the product below acquisition cost.

MAC. The MAC is the maximum allowable cost, which is the federally set reimbursement rate for generic drugs used in the Medicaid system. Many other payers use MAC systems as well. The federal MAC is also called the FFP, which stands for federal financial participation. It is set at 150% of the lowest generally available price for generics.

Manufacturer's List Price. As the name implies, the list price is a price that has been published by a manufacturer. Many manufacturers make actual list prices available only to wholesalers, providing a catalog that contains AWPs to the nonwholesale trade (see Ex-Factory Price).

Net Price. Also known as "landed price," this is the price, or revenue, realized by a manufacturer after all discounts have been granted.

Net Profit (Margin). Net profit margin is the difference in selling price and all costs associated with doing business, allocated on a per-unit basis.

OBRA 90. The Omnibus Budget Reconciliation Act of 1990, a law drafted by the Senate Committee on Aging, requires manufacturers to pay rebates to state and federal governments for products used by Medicaid recipients.

Rebate. A rebate is a retroactive discount that is paid to a customer after that customer has purchased the product from a wholesaler or retailer. The rebate allows the manufacturer to offer a lower price to some customers without taking on the burden of special distribution mechanisms.

Standard Cost. The product costing system used by most pharmaceutical firms is called "standard costing" or "fully absorbed cost." With this system, in addition to the variable costs such as ingredients, packaging, and direct labor, a portion of fixed cost (overhead) is allocated to each product and package. This cost is allocated on the basis of forecasts made at the beginning of the fiscal year. Such a system assures that, when unit volume increases, the incremental cost of a unit will decline, while the incremental cost of a product with a declining sales trend will increase significantly. It is not uncommon for half or more of a product's standard cost to consist of this fixed cost allocation.

Wholesale Acquisition Price (WAC). This term is used by some publishers of pricing data to denote the ex-factory charge, before discounts, to the wholesaler.

WHAT IS A PHARMACEUTICAL PRICE?

Although it might appear otherwise, given the number of sources of drug pricing information, comparing or computing the prices of drugs is not straightforward. Differences in the manner in which various prices are set and used render many comparisons virtually meaningless.

Different prices are charged to and by different members of the distribution channels used for pharmaceuticals. Some prices are set using traditional methods, while others are set according to competitive conditions. Even within the same pharmacy several different pricing methods will be used, depending on a number of factors. Figure 1 outlines typical approaches to pricing both branded and generic products in a retail pharmacy. These and other retail pricing tactics are discussed below. In the hospital setting, different rules and methods are used. The flow of prices within hospitals is presented in Figure 2.

As Figures 1 and 2 demonstrate, the price of a pharmaceutical product depends on a number of factors. Prices and costs of drugs vary on many levels and depend upon factors such as the location of drug administration, the relative commercial success of the agent, and the type of manufacturer supplying the drug, to name just a few.

AWP

The AWP is the most common figure used for drug price comparisons. This figure is a vestige of a drug distribution system that disappeared in the early 1980s. Until the early 1980s, there were several hundred small, independent drug wholesalers, each operating regionally. Due to the inefficiencies of such a fragmented system, the operating costs were quite high. The average markup above cost by wholesalers to their retail customers (primarily pharmacies) was 20% to 25%, depending on the manufacturer.

FIGURE 1. Flow of Price for a Retail-Dispensed Outpatient Drug.

Ex-Factory Price (Wholesaler Cost) => Wholesaler Price (Retailer Cost) => Retail Price (Patient/Payer Cost)

Branded Pharmaceutical

Ex-Factory Price (Wholesaler Cost) => Wholesaler Price (Retailer Cost) => Retail Price (Patient/Payer Cost)
$10 less cash discount (2%)   => "Cost" ($10) + 2% to 5%   => "Cost" (AWP, $12) + fee = $17

Generic Pharmaceutical

Ex-Factory Price (Wholesaler Cost) => Wholesaler Price (Retailer Cost) => Retail Price (Patient/Payer Cost)
$1.00 less cash discount (2%)   => "Cost" ($1.00) + 2% to 5%   => "Cost" (AWP, $3.00) + fee = $8

OR

$1.00 less cash discount (2%)   => "Cost" ($1.00) + 2% to 5%   => Brand Price less 30% = $ 11.90

FIGURE 2. Examples of the Flow of Price for a Hospital-Dispensed Drug.

Ex-Factory Price (Wholesaler Cost)	=>	Discount ("Chargeback") (Hospital Cost)	=>	Hospital Price (Patient/Payer Cost)
Branded Pharmaceutical				
Ex-Factory Price (Wholesaler Cost)	=>	"Chargeback" (Hospital Cost)	=>	Hospital Price (Patient/Payer Cost)
$10/100 doses, less cash discount (2%)	=>	"Cost" ($10) – $2 "Chargeback"	=>	Fixed Charge per dose $2.25 × 100 = $225
Generic Pharmaceutical				
Ex-Factory Price (Wholesaler Cost)	=>	Wholesaler Price (Hospital Cost)	=>	Hospital Price (Patient/Payer Cost)
$10/100 doses, less cash discount (2%)	=>	"Cost" ($10)	=>	Fixed Charge per dose $2.25 × 100 = $225

While most pharmaceutical manufacturers used a wholesaler-only method of distribution to the retail class of trade, a significant number of large firms, including Upjohn, Merck, and Squibb, had invested in their own distribution networks and preferred direct sales over the use of wholesalers. By convention, wholesalers added 20% to the price of products from companies following a wholesaler-only policy while adding 25% to the prices of products from those companies who chose to "compete" with the wholesalers.

In the late 1970s and early 1980s, several wholesale drug companies began to acquire smaller competitors. Two companies in particular, Bergen Brunswig Company and McKesson Drug, expanded significantly. Both became national in scope during this period, resulting in the existence of fewer than 90 separate wholesale drug companies in the United States today.

The expansion of major wholesale firms also concentrated competition. Before consolidation, most wholesalers had little or no competition within their trade areas, so there was no pressure to reduce their markups. As consolidation in the industry increased, major companies began competing for the same business, resulting in price competition.

Additionally, during the 1980s, prices charged by manufacturers began to increase. This allowed the wholesalers to practice arbitrage—buying drugs in anticipation of price increases, then selling their inventory at the new, higher prices. These combined forces brought the average wholesale markup in the early 1990s to roughly 2.5%, significantly lower than the markup implied by the published AWP.

Wholesalers have two different methods of pricing to the retailers: AWP minus and cost plus. As the names imply, one method begins with the published AWP while the other ignores this figure. In recent years, cost-plus pricing has become the norm for most wholesalers. Price reporting services, however, still rely upon the AWP because, until recently, many companies published only that figure (often called the "suggested price to pharmacy"). The AWP, while not the cost paid by retailers, still provides the basis for much retail pricing, with retailers euphemistically referring to the difference between their actual cost and the AWP as "earned discount." This tradition is so ingrained that a retailer that sells a product at

AWP, which is roughly 18% above the retailer's cost, refers to this price as a loss leader.

This situation is more pronounced with generic drugs. Many generic companies have taken advantage of this use of AWP by substantially inflating their published AWPs. The most dramatic move was in 1989, when Geneva Generics increased some AWPs by over 1000% while decreasing selling prices. Soon many other generic companies instituted similar policies. This system allows a retailer to acquire a drug at a low cost ($2.50 per 100 tablets, for example) while relying on a published AWP ($20.00 or more) for its own pricing. It is not uncommon that the $25.00 retail price for a generic drug renders a gross profit well above $20.00 for the retailer. It is also common for the AWP of a generic product to remain stable while the actual selling price declines.

Table 1 shows the wide disparity between actual selling prices and published AWPs for several pharmaceutical products. It is obvious that AWP is not an accurate measure of the prices manufacturers charge. It must also be noted that not all generic products will

TABLE 1. The Difference Between Costs and AWP for Packages of 100 Tablets.

PRODUCT	Ex-Factory Price	AWP	Percentage Difference
Tylenol with Codeine #3	$25.93	$31.13	20%
Mutual acetaminophen w/ codeine 300-30	$3.94	$10.00	174%
Tagamet 300mg	$77.36	$96.70	20%
URL cimetidine 300mg	$29.93	$76.40	155%
Xanax 0.5mg	$61.86	$77.66	25%
URL alprazolam 0.5mg	$4.81	$61.12	1,168%

SOURCE: Medispan Price-Check Data Base, February, 1996.

be priced similarly. Some, in fact, use the more traditional method of a 20% markup to reach an AWP. This can be a handicap for generic companies choosing this method because retailers often use the AWP as the starting point for many pricing decisions and an artificially high AWP provides the retailer with greater profits.

Retail Prices

Retail pharmacies also use several different methods for pricing their products. Because many, if not most, retail pricing methods use the AWP as a starting point, it should be obvious that the profitability for different products can vary widely. Table 2 presents data from an audit of retail prescription prices that is performed regularly by IMS America. As in Table 1, AWP is not the best measure for price comparisons between products or a good indicator of actual prices paid.

While the AWP provides the basis for much retail pricing, many

TABLE 2. Typical Retail Pricing Approaches (prices per tab/cap).

PRODUCT	Pharmacy Net Cost	AWP	Average Retail Price	Difference
Prozac 20mg	$1.863	$2.201	$2.14	14.9%
Zoloft 50mg	$1.655	$1.941	$2.11	27.5%
Pamelor 25mg	$0.784	$0.910	$1.10	40.3%
nortriptyline (Schein) 25mg	$0.159	$0.765	$0.62	289.9%
Mevacor 20mg	$1.696	$2.084	$1.86	9.7%
Lescol 20mg	$0.916	$1.064	$1.17	27.7%
amoxicillin (Biocraft) 500mg	$0.069	$0.210	$0.45	552.2%
Augmentin 500mg	$2.247	$2.882	$2.98	32.6%

SOURCE: National Prescription Audit®, 1st Quarter, 1996, Copyright IMS America, Ltd. All Rights Reserved.

other factors intervene in the determination of the price of a specific product. Generally, the two most influential factors are the relative commercial success of the agent and its duration of use. Each of these factors exerts a different effect.

Commercial Success. Commercial success influences the retail price because high-selling agents are often featured by discounters in their promotion. A product such as Mevacor® (lovastatin), for cholesterol control, or Vasotec® (enalapril), for hypertension, will often be used by retailers as a loss leader to enhance store traffic. High sales levels of these products, together with the likelihood that a patient taking the agent is also using other medications, allows the retailer to forego normal profits for that agent and make a return on other patient purchases.

Products that are less successful commercially will often receive significantly higher markups. A general rule of thumb is that pharmaceutical products will receive a "full retail" markup, which can range from 20% to 100% above AWP, until they have proven themselves in the marketplace. Once a product achieves sales of roughly $50 million annually and has a refill prescription rate above 50%, the typical retailer will begin to price the product "competitively," where the markup ranges between 5% and 15% above AWP. For extremely successful products–those whose sales exceed $200 million annually–retailers often choose the loss leader pricing tactic, which averages between 10% below and 10% above AWP.

This is an important consideration for the manufacturer about to launch a new agent into a successful market. Because newer products will be priced at full retail and successful products are likely to be used as loss leaders, pricing a new product, at ex-factory, precisely the same way as a major competitor could result in the patient paying as much as *40% more* for the new product. Even if the new product is priced 20% below the market leader, it could be more expensive for the patient until it has achieved sales over the $200 million mark.

Duration of Use. Duration of use has a major influence on retail pricing because the retailer knows a medication for an acute condition, such as minor pain or infection, is less likely to be a shopping item, a product for which a patient will seek out the lowest price. For chronic conditions, however, patients can anticipate the purchase and shop for lower prices. As such, the markup on chronic medications will range from slightly below AWP to 25% above it, depending on the market success of the product, while acute medications–those with a refill rate below 50%–can be priced as high as AWP plus 50% or more.

Another factor that affects the retail price is the store type. A chain drugstore is likely to set prices below that of an independent community pharmacy because its volume will allow such actions. A mass merchandiser such as Wal-Mart or K-Mart will sell at prices below those of the chains because its pharmacies are seen as traffic builders for the stores. It is not uncommon for the mass retailers to establish policies forbidding their pharmacies to operate at a profit because higher prices might result in attracting fewer customers to the store.

Retail prices are often determined on the basis of the most common package size for a product, usually packages of 100. If a product is available in a larger package (e.g., 500s) and that package is available at a discount when compared with the package of 100, the retail customer, or repackager, will buy the product in 500s but sell it at the 100 count price. This issue is of great importance because it widens the gap between the manufacturer's average selling price and the price paid by the patient.

Hospital Costs and Prices

Many hospitals and managed care systems receive favorable pricing from pharmaceutical companies. Some of these discounts are meant to encourage physician use in hospitals in hope that this use will spill over into physicians' private practices. Teaching hospitals also receive favorable prices in hope that interns and residents trained on a product will continue to use it once they enter private practice.

These approaches have resulted in significant price competition in institutional sectors. Discounts ranging from 10% to 80% below list prices (which are themselves 16% to 20% below AWP) are not uncommon in most hospitals.

The hospitals, in turn, apply simple methodologies in pricing their products. Oral agents are customarily priced by the dose. The national average is roughly $2.50 per tablet or capsule for products with acquisition costs below $1.50 per dose. A similarly high markup is applied to more expensive agents. Thus, acetaminophen with codeine, which the hospital can purchase for less than 1¢ per tablet, would be priced at $2.50 per tablet on the patient's bill. For a full day's therapy of 2 tablets every 4 hours (12 tablets), the bill could be as high as $30.00 (1).

Injectable agents, which may also be discounted, are priced in a fashion that incorporates AWP and the time and materials required for administration. As with outpatient medications, the role of AWP is to exaggerate the acquisition cost and allow for maximum reimbursement in fee-for-service situations.

Prime Vendors and Group Purchasers

Recall that in the 1980s drug wholesalers became larger and fewer and much more competitive. Wholesalers began to expand their customer bases and to pursue more business with hospitals and other nonretail accounts. At the same time, hospitals banded together in buying groups. Several hospitals pooled their business and, with significantly more buying power, were able to secure lower prices from many manufacturers.

Such a system worked well with small numbers of hospitals, but as the number of hospitals within a group increased, it became nearly impossible to keep track of the transactions between hospitals and different pharmaceutical companies. By placing a wholesaler between hospitals and drug companies, one entity could then be responsible for tracking and coordinating purchases. This wholesaler, then, became the prime vendor to the hospitals, and all (or most) pharmaceutical purchases by the member hospitals were made through a single wholesaler. This posed a problem, however, because hospitals had negotiated prices that were below those available to the wholesaler. A solution was reached with the development of the chargeback, defined earlier in this section.

The prime vendor usually works for a standard markup, often cost plus 2%. Like manufacturers, wholesalers must compete and submit bids to gain the business of the buying group. Although the 2% markup on a large amount of business can generate substantial revenues, the wholesaler has another source of revenue in the cash discount. Because the discount is paid for timely payment, it is not reflected on invoices, and most prime vendor contracts allow the wholesaler to keep such discounts as long as the costs to the buying group are not increased.

Thus, a wholesale prime vendor receives a 2% cash discount, sells the product to the hospital group, and receives another 2% fee for the service. While this can be quite lucrative for the wholesaler, manufacturers–especially those who offer large discounts (charge-backs) to hospitals–can find themselves making little profit on some transactions. Consider a product with a list price (WAC or ex-factory) of $10.00 that required a discount of 80% to secure the hospital business. By tracking the various prices of this product as it flowed through the system, we would see the effects as shown in Table 3. In this case, the $2.00 contract price nets the pharmaceutical company $1.80 in sales, the wholesaler earns $0.24 on a $2.00 product (12%), and the hospital has a net cost of $2.04.

NOW, WHAT WAS THE PRICE OF THAT DRUG?

To recap the major messages of this chapter, let's look at a hypothetical product that can be used in both outpatient and inpatient settings. Among the factors to consider are:

- The product is still under patent protection, sells approximately $125 million per year, and is taken/administered twice daily. Refill prescriptions constitute roughly 50% of its total outpatient business.
- The current ex-factory price is $30.00 per 100 tablets, with a 500 count package available for $140.00. Because the product is sold only to wholesalers, AWP markup is 20%.
- There are a few competing compounds in the same class, so discounts are believed to be necessary to secure hospital business. Due to the requirements of long-term contracting, the current contract price to hospitals is 25% below ex-factory price.

Let's follow this product as it leaves the shipping docks and examine the pricing and profit flow, as presented in Table 4.

The product the manufacturer priced at $30.00 for a package of

TABLE 3. Pricing Flow for a Hospital Product.

Ex-Factory Price	Cash Discount	Wholesaler Net Cost	Price to Hospital	Chargeback	Net Price to Manufacturer
$10.00	$0.20	$9.80	$2.04	$8.00	$1.80

TABLE 4. Review of Pricing Flow.

		Retail Customer		Hospital	
		100 Count	500 Count	100 Count	500 Count
AWP		$36.00	$168.00	$36.00	$128.00
Wholesaler Transactions:	Ex-Factory Price:	$30.00	$140.00	$30.00	$140.00
	Cash Discount	$0.60	$2.80	$0.60	$2.80
Chargeback:	(Hospital only)			$7.50	$35.00
	Wholesaler Net Cost	$29.40	$137.20	$21.90	$102.20
Price:	Retail (Cost + 3%) Hospital (25% discount + 2%)	$30.90	$144.20	$22.95	$107.10
Wholesaler Profit:		$1.50 (5%)	$7.00 (5%)	$1.05 (4.8%)	$4.90 (4.8%)
Retail/Hospital Transactions Price:	Retail, Rx of 100 (AWP + $5.00)	$41.00	$41.00/100 ($205.00)		
	Hospital 100 doses @ $2.50/dose			$250.00	$1,250.00
Profit (as % of sales)		$10.10 (24.6%)	$67.80 (33.1%)	$227.05 (90.8%)	$1,142.90 (91.4%)

100 tablets and \$140.00 for a package of 500 tablets, then, has several other prices, depending on the customer and specific point in the distribution channel. As shown in Table 4, the prices range from \$21.90 to \$250.00 for a single package size.

The complexities of pharmaceutical pricing—with their conditions, discounts, and tactical schemes—render simple analyses useless. When discussing the prices of pharmaceuticals, then, it is important to ask *which price?*

REFERENCE

1. Kolassa EM. Guidance for clinicians in discerning the prices of pharmaceutical agents. J Pain Symptom Manage 1994;9(4):235-43.

Price Decision Making

INTRODUCTION

Pricing decisions are reached in a number of ways, using a varied range of considerations, types of information, and internal processes. Each pricing decision is unique, depending on the company, the medication, and the external factors that affect both. In this section, the factors that should be considered when making pricing decisions are discussed. There is no one "best" or "right" manner in which to set prices, but there are a group of considerations and processes that appear to offer a company the best chance of making informed pricing decisions.

KEY FACTORS IN THE PRICING DECISION

The pharmaceutical pricing question most frequently asked by those observing (or criticizing) the pharmaceutical industry is: How are drug prices set? Many self-proclaimed experts have offered answers to this question, usually armed with summaries of financial statements that document the way in which pharmaceutical companies spend their revenues. This financial information is not, in fact, related to the pricing of a new medication. Attempts to reduce the pricing process to a simple formula not only are misleading but also reflect an absolute lack of knowledge about the pricing of medicines.

It is unlikely that any two pharmaceutical companies set prices

[Haworth co-indexing entry note]: "Price Decision Making." Kolassa, E. M. (Mick). Co-published simultaneously in *Journal of Pharmaceutical Marketing Practice* (The Pharmaceutical Products Press, an imprint of The Haworth Press, Inc.) Vol. 1, No. 1 (#1), 1997, pp. 45-61; and: *Elements of Pharmaceutical Pricing* (E. M. (Mick) Kolassa) The Pharmaceutical Products Press, an imprint of The Haworth Press, Inc., 1997, pp. 45-61. Single or multiple copies of this article are available for a fee from The Haworth Document Delivery Service [1-800-342-9678, 9:00 a.m. - 5:00 p.m. (EST). E-mail address: getinfo@haworth.com].

using the same thought processes–or even consider the same issues when establishing a price. Moreover, it is unlikely that a single company would price any two different products in the same way, given differences in markets, timing, market entry dynamics, and other environmental factors. This lack of singularity, which critics may question, is actually quite appropriate. No two companies have exactly the same needs, philosophies, or resources, and no two separate products will be marketed using precisely the same strategy, even if sold by the same company. These basic differences demand different pricing criteria and different prices.

The pricing of pharmaceutical products, as with the pricing of any product or service, should be market based. Contrary to the widely held notion that pricing is simply a matter of adding up costs and establishing a markup, pricing experts agree that costs help establish a price floor but the market provides most of the information for the pricing decision. As competition within pharmaceutical markets, especially price-related competition, heats up, the need for market-based pricing will continue to grow.

There are some general rules, or considerations, that should be included in every pharmaceutical pricing decision. These factors, presented in Figure 1, must be addressed, either formally through adherence to a company policy or informally by a product manager or other individual charged with developing a pricing recommendation. The failure to address these factors can contribute to many pricing missteps in pharmaceutical markets.

FIGURE 1. General Factors to Consider When Setting a Pharmaceutical Price

1. The prices, product features, and past actions of the competition
2. Specific patient characteristics
3. The economic and social value of the therapy itself
4. The decision-making criteria of prescribers and those who influence that decision
5. Characteristics of the disease treated by the medication
6. Company needs, in terms of market position, revenue, and other issues
7. Company abilities, including available budgets and willingness to support the product
8. The current and anticipated environment for insurance reimbursement
9. The public policy environment

To further complicate the process, it is likely that the elements of this simple model will vary greatly among different companies and company affiliates, as local variations in health care delivery, reimbursement, and regulations compound the problems. Still, these issues must be investigated and addressed.

COMPETITION

Typically, the first pieces of information a company gathers when arriving at a price recommendation are the prices of competing drugs. If a new product is to be launched into a therapeutic area that is already served by one or more agents, the prices of those agents should provide initial guidance in price selection. Which prices to use for this analysis, such as ex-factory prices, discount prices, or price per dose/per day of therapy/per package/per course of therapy, will depend upon the perspective of the analysis and the product under study. Generally, list (or ex-factory) prices for a comparable unit of therapy, whether that is a single day's therapy for a chronic disorder or a complete course of therapy for an acute treatment, are an appropriate place to begin. Discounts and other considerations are tactical in nature, and the first steps in any analysis of initial pricing should be focused on strategy.

In addition to the current prices of competitive agents, the price histories of products in this class should be examined to assess any recent changes in the price positions of the various products. Anticipated competitive product launches must also be considered. The range of prices for branded products in this market, from highest to lowest, should also be examined. If the price levels seem to be related to relative market success of the agents (e.g., those with the highest market shares seem to have prices that are either higher or lower than their less successful competitors), this could indicate the presence or absence of significant price sensitivity. High-priced market leaders imply little or no price sensitivity, while lower-priced leaders may imply the opposite.

The prices of other products sold by the major competitors and recent entrants in this market should also be investigated to determine whether their pricing in this market reflects a company pricing policy or a deliberate pricing strategy for this specific market. If the prices reflect a departure from a firm's typical approach to pricing, that may be a signal that price sensitivity is at work in this market, or at least that the company believes that is the case.

Other competitive factors that must be assessed at this stage are the level of promotion by other agents, their rates of growth, and the extent of discounting in price-sensitive markets such as managed care and hospitals. Here again, the level of discounting must be compared with the success of the products in those discounted markets. High levels of promotional spending in a market make it difficult for a new agent to break through. If the decision makers can be swayed with a low-price appeal, markets with significant promotional spending may be good targets for a low-price strategy–if you can determine how low the price must be to gain prescribers' attention. This approach usually requires high levels of spending as well.

Low levels of promotional spending imply a satisfied or mature market, which may be less responsive to low-price positioning. Conversely, it may imply a mature market with little true competition and patients with unmet needs. In such markets, a new agent that offers improvements over those currently available can often command a premium with no negative effect on prescribing levels. In many cases, products launched at discounts were perceived by physicians to be priced at premiums because of the improvements in quality; the prescribers assumed that the better product cost more (1). In such cases, prescriber decision making plays a major role in the pricing decision.

Relative market share, compared with price levels, is also a telling statistic. In markets where the leading products are also those with the lowest prices, it may mean that the markets are extremely price sensitive. Figure 2 portrays this relationship graphically. The market leader is also the product with the highest price, and the lowest priced agent holds the lowest share of market. In this case, one can conclude that the market is not price sensitive.

In Figure 3, the opposite holds true. The market leader is also the product that has the lowest price. Note that this does not automatically imply that the market is price sensitive, only that the competitors appear to be price sensitive. But there are indications that the market is aware of and responds to price differences.

FIGURE 2. Graph of Price Sensitivity of Market, Nonsensitive Market.

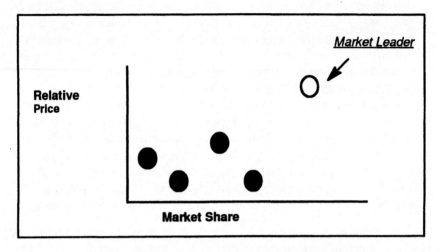

FIGURE 3. Graph of a Potentially Sensitive Market.

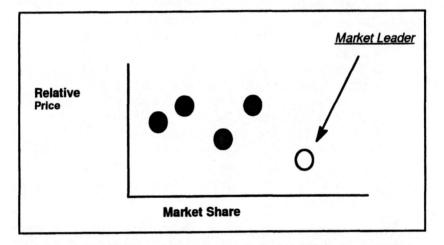

The importance of competitive analysis in pricing cannot be overstated. It has been suggested by many researchers that the pricing and presence of competitors, together with the uniqueness or therapeutic value of the new product, are the major determinants of launch prices. Reekie, in his manuscript "Pricing New Pharmaceutical Products," found that the price levels of current competitors and the anticipation of future competitors were the driving factors in setting prices for pharmaceuticals (2). New entrants that offered significant benefits over current competitors were consistently priced above the prevailing prices in the therapeutic class. Those products offering little or no therapeutic advantage tended to be priced at or below prevailing levels.

An interesting finding of Reekie's study, however, was that, even for unique products offering improvements, those that had close or superior competitors entering the market within two years of their launch tended to be priced lower than those that anticipated little or no competition from new products in the near future. The general rule can be seen graphically in Figure 4. The rule portrayed in Figure 4 is a simple application of the three basic pricing strategies:

1. *Skimming.* The product, anticipating little direct competition, is priced above prevailing levels to maximize profits. Prilosec[®], the first proton pump inhibitor, was priced in this manner, substantially above the price levels of the H_2 antagonists.

2. *Parity.* The product is viewed internally as being little or no different from current competitors and is priced equivalent to the prevailing levels. The nonsedating antihistamine Claritin[®] and the ACE inhibitor Accupril[®] were priced at parity to the market leaders at the times of their launches.

3. *Penetration.* A product is viewed as equal to or slightly inferior to current or anticipated offerings and is priced below prevailing levels in hopes of gaining market share with its low price or of erecting a barrier to entry for anticipated future competitors. Lescol[®] appears to be the only pharmaceutical product to have successfully employed a penetration pricing strategy.

These strategies also depend on other factors, such as the needs and abilities of the company, the sensitivity of the specific market segment to price levels, and the therapeutic value of the product itself. Thus, the considerations presented here are not discrete entities to be considered separately, but a complex system that must be evaluated as a whole.

Reekie and others have noted that, although it appears that most

FIGURE 4. Competitive Considerations in Pricing.

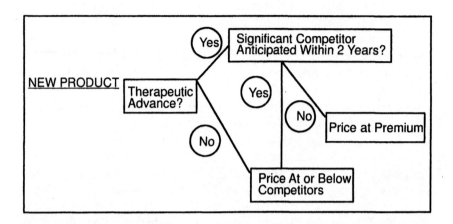

pharmaceutical markets are not price sensitive, most companies act–and price–as though they believe they are sensitive. The lack of responsiveness to the deep discounts in many markets in the U.S. implies that:

- These markets do not respond to price.
- The companies marketing many of the products act as though they believe the markets are responsive to price.

Belief in price sensitivity, as opposed to an objective measurement of price sensitivity, appears to have led many pharmaceutical companies to underprice their products. A "me-too" product priced at a 30% discount and achieving a market share of 2% to 5%, which can be expected of most such products regardless of price, implies that the 30% discount represents an opportunity cost to the company of nearly 50%. This means that a price 50% above that charged may have delivered the same level of unit sales as the lower price, but with significantly greater dollar sales and profits.

PATIENT CHARACTERISTICS

Although in many markets the patient bears no direct financial burden, this is not the case in all markets. In markets without universal coverage for pharmaceuticals, the patients who will be the final users of a new agent must be considered in the pricing decision. In the U.S., for example, a great proportion of the elderly population has no third-party coverage for medications and must pay for them out of pocket. If the bulk of the patient population who will use a product is elderly, their ability to afford the product, in addition to other medications, must always be considered. Although a product may seem relatively inexpensive at $1.50 per day, the total cost can be prohibitive for a patient on a fixed income taking 3 or 4 such prescriptions on a daily basis.

Such considerations are not simply altruism, although there is room for compassion in every strategy. The fact is, patients who are unable to afford a medication will often not take it. Compliance, both with the daily dosing and the length of therapy, is a growing concern and a source of significant unrealized revenue (3, 4). It is not uncommon for 50% of patients prescribed a medication for a chronic disorder that is relatively asymptomatic to drop out in the first year (5, 6). How much of this is due to failure to understand the importance of compliance versus inability to afford the medication is not yet known, but if a significant proportion of this can be eliminated with a lower price, the product may earn more with a lower price than a higher one (7).

Some patient groups are highly organized and able to exert political and economic pressure on a company. The areas of mental health, Parkinson's disease, HIV, and cancer all have active support groups that are playing a growing role in therapy selection. The degree of patient involvement in therapy decisions appears to be growing across most major therapeutic categories, and the market power of these groups must play an ever-growing role in pricing decisions.

Yet even in markets where patients are shielded from the financial consequences of medication use, patients can, and do, play a role in the adoption of many agents, and their demand for some products can provide price flexibility. In the U.S., the most price-sensitive buyer may be the giant HMO Kaiser Permanente, a staff-model HMO with many restrictive policies and the ability to limit drug use. Schering Plough refused to grant Kaiser the major price concessions the HMO demanded, and Kaiser then refused to list the

Schering antihistamine Claritin on its formulary, denying Schering access to Kaiser patients. In doing so, Kaiser also denied its patients access to Claritin, and the protests from patients were overwhelming. In the end, Schering was able to get Claritin on the Kaiser formulary without granting major discounts. In many such cases where patients are very involved in treatment of their disorders (diseases such as diabetes, asthma, allergy, and many others), patient pull-through may enable the company to command higher prices than pricing authorities may be initially willing to grant. It is wise to examine this possibility when the launch of appropriate medications is anticipated and perhaps wait for patients to demand reimbursement for the product.

VALUE OF THERAPY

It is wise to begin economic as well as clinical studies early in the clinical development process. Among the first pieces of "outcomes" work should be a financial profile of the disease for which the agent is being investigated. Such an analysis allows the fitting of the agent into this financial profile to determine its potential effect on the cost of treatment.

Ideally, any new agent will help to reduce the cost of treatment, especially if there are already pharmacologic therapies available. In theory, the value of a new agent is equal to the cost reduction it provides. Should the use of a new agent reduce the cost of treatment of the disorder by $1,000 per year, before considering the price for the product, its "economic value" is $1,000.

If this new agent has significant clinical or quality of life advantages over current therapy and would provide better overall patient care and outcomes for the same cost, pricing the product to capture its entire economic value of $1,000 would be appropriate. Unfortunately, though, pricing is not always this straightforward and certainly not this simple, and many in the marketplace appear to resist the use of such information in product adoption decisions. A study by Kolassa and Smith, for example, found that hospital pharmacy directors in the U.S. were incapable of fully understanding and processing the results of pharmacoeconomic studies and, although they believed these studies would become important in the future, found them to be of little value today (8).

It is unlikely that any new agent could be documented to reduce costs by a precise figure. Instead, savings ranges are the more likely result, due to regulatory, patient, and provider differences. These ranges do, however, provide a range for pricing as well and can certainly help to establish a price ceiling, or maximum reasonable price. The company's own costs and margin requirements, based on unit cost or standard cost figures, would provide the price floor.

Given the focus on and need for health care reform and cost containment, an agent that can deliver documented cost savings should (in ideal circumstances) be well received. But one must look to other issues as well to assure the acceptance of this argument. The reimbursement and public policy environments will both affect this.

THE DECISION-MAKING PROCESS

The specific decision maker for the use of the agent plays a large role in the effectiveness of any pricing approach. Products that will be used primarily on an in-patient basis will be subjected to significant price scrutiny, as the institutional market is, perhaps, the most price sensitive single pharmaceutical market. Because of the influence of multiple decision makers, including pharmacy directors and hospital administrators, the cost of any new agent will be considered carefully before the agent is adopted. Several studies have shown that clinical pharmacists, through various outreach and educational efforts, can bring about a significant change in physician prescribing behavior (9-12). Lazarus and Smith (1988) reported that 52% of pharmacist interventions in response to reviews of prescriptions written in an Alabama medical center resulted in changes in medications (13). That pharmacists can—and do—intervene in and influence the prescribing decision, then, is well established. Their potential role in the use of a new product must be seriously considered.

In the outpatient setting, the practitioner can often choose therapies without regard to cost. Not that an outpatient drug is not subject to price sensitivity. The growth of managed care in the U.S., local fundholders in the U.K., local budgets in Germany, and other initiatives elsewhere have the potential to increase the level of price sensitivity over time.

Primary care physicians are often more risk averse than their specialized colleagues and are unlikely to adopt a new medication as rapidly as a neurologist or a cardiologist (14). New agents whose use will be limited to specialists are unlikely to come under any price scrutiny by the prescriber, since specialists tend to be less concerned with (or aware of) the costs of the treatments they order. It stands to reason that they would be less likely to receive feedback on drug costs from patients than primary care physicians, who see patients more regularly and are more likely to operate under systems that force them to bear (or share) the costs of their decisions.

Unfortunately, another consideration in this area is the potential for competition by and with prescribing physicians. There are several cases in which the use of a new agent is a direct threat to a procedure that one or more physician specialties rely upon. Routine use of some thrombolytic agents has been resisted by vascular surgeons, who may perceive the drugs as threats to their own livelihoods. Studies comparing thrombolytic use with vascular surgery are interesting in that those performed by vascular surgeons tend to conclude that surgery is not only safer and more effective but also less costly than the use of thrombolytics alone. Studies performed by radiologists and other nonsurgeons, however, show the opposite. The situation is, as yet, unresolved, and several more studies will be done to clarify the issue. The lack of resolution has allowed many decision makers to assume, without benefit of adequate documentation, that the prices of thrombolytics are too high.

DISEASE CHARACTERISTICS

The characteristics of the disease itself can provide some of the most valuable guidance in establishing a pricing strategy. Experience shows that disorders of an acute nature, such as minor infectious diseases and pain due to injury, tend not to be accompanied by price sensitivity. Patients receiving a prescription for an antibiotic or analgesic usually receive no refills and often do not follow up with the physician. This appears to hold true even in situations where the patient pays the full cost of the prescription. For chronic disorders, however, patients pay the price every month and often complain to the prescribing physician about the cost of medications. In the U.S., retail pharmacists, for competitive reasons, usually apply lower markups to chronically used medications than to those for acute therapy (15).

Research indicates that there could be an additional dimension to this—that of the symptoms of the disease (16). Physicians appear to overestimate the cost of medications that treat chronic, asymptomatic diseases, such as hypertension, and to underestimate the cost of medications that treat more symptomatic disorders such as arthritis and acute infections. It has been postulated that this is due to the type of patient feedback the physician receives. A patient paying $1.00 each day to treat a disease he or she doesn't feel, such as hypertension, should be expected to complain of the cost more than patients whose NSAID is relieving the pain of arthritis and allowing them to lead a more normal life.

Thus, it is likely that the prescriber will overestimate the cost of your product if it treats a relatively asymptomatic chronic disorder and generates a large amount of negative feedback. This overestimation may result in fewer prescriptions. Figure 5 portrays the general findings of a study of physicians' price estimates.

THE REIMBURSEMENT ENVIRONMENT

In highly regulated health care systems, such as many European systems, reimbursement and pricing are nearly synonymous: the price is what the agency is willing to pay. Care must be exercised in dealing with these agencies, and it is worthwhile to remember that success depends on being a price maker and not a price taker in such markets. Understanding the needs and motives of the reimbursement authorities and their history with your firm and others often determines the difference between receiving a good price or a not-so-good one.

The reimbursement environment must always be considered. Agents used in the inpatient setting are often reimbursed as part of the total hospital charge. Costly agents, or those perceived as such, could be restricted in their use, either by the hospital or by the insurers. Many agents are placed on prior authorization lists in

FIGURE 5. Physicians' Price Estimates and the Nature of the Disorder.

	SYMPTOMATIC	ASYMPTOMATIC
A C U T E	Tendency to underestimate actual cost. Average estimate 35% below actual. Examples: antibiotics, analgesics.	N/A
C H R O N I C	Generally the most accurate estimates. Examples: NSAIDs, antiulcerants.	Tendency to overestimate, often by 100% or more. Examples: Antihypertensives, hormone replacement.

SOURCE: Kolassa EM. Physicians' perceptions of prescription drug prices: their accuracy and effect on the prescribing decision. J Res Pharm Econ 1995; 6(1): 23-37.

hospitals and their use restricted to certain physicians. While these situations are not yet routine, economic studies that support the price and reimbursement assistance programs may relieve some pressures and allow a price that is higher than would otherwise be accepted by the market.

Insurance reimbursement status has been shown to affect drug product selection in the in-patient setting. Some researchers have found that patients with comprehensive coverage receive more–and more expensive–medications than those with less adequate insurance coverage (17).

Finally, a major consideration in the reimbursement environment is the effect of managed care formularies. Securing placement on these formularies has often required discounting from list price. Should a significant portion of the potential market be subject to such formulary management–and this portion is growing rapidly–setting a price that is acceptable in the "open" market may render the product overpriced in managed care settings. Appropriate discounts to some segments may be useful in these cases, but the legislative and judicial moves favoring uniform pricing for pharmaceuticals may make this more difficult in the near future. It may be wise to establish the appropriate price for managed care and use this price for all market segments.

COMPANY NEEDS

While the cost of goods and company-established minimum selling margins play a role in the establishment of a price floor, other company-specific issues must also be addressed. New research investment or activities that are expected to require significant amounts of funding might well necessitate the charging of a higher price for agents about to be launched, providing the higher price would not negatively affect the sales of the product.

Conversely, a new agent may be seen as simply providing the company with experience in a therapeutic category prior to the introduction of an agent that is felt to be superior some years later. In this case, a low-price strategy on an agent without significant advantages could allow the company to develop this experience and important relationships with prescribers and key thought leaders in this market.

Finally, an innovative pricing strategy that may offer savings, guarantees, or some other feature could result in positive press coverage for the company. This may be seen as valuable for investor or customer relations.

COMPANY ABILITIES

The ability and willingness of the company to support the pricing strategy must always be considered. A high price in a sensitive market requires significant resources by way of economic studies and, often, senior management time to alleviate much of the price resistance. Similarly, a low-priced strategy in an outpatient market is likely to cost more in promotional expenses than parity pricing if the strategy is to be successful. This is because physicians, as previously mentioned, tend not to respond to low-priced appeals. A successful low-priced approach requires significant promotional expenditures to saturate the market with the message that the product is less costly and to induce physicians to consider cost.

Prescribing physicians do not actively seek out price information and often do not respond to low prices even when they are aware of them (18). A penetration strategy requires greater promotional coverage and more creative selling messages to instill a sense of economic responsibility (or guilt) in prescribers than the approach of simply charging whatever the competition charges.

Whether the company chooses a price that is significantly above or below the prevailing prices in the market, top management must be willing to spend the time and the money necessary to support the pricing strategy.

PUBLIC POLICY CONSIDERATIONS

Last, but certainly not least, is the public policy environment. In the foreseeable future, a company must consider the responses and actions of government officials and patient advocates when setting a price. Criticism by one of these individuals, no matter how unfounded, can result in severe limits on the potential success of a new drug. Once a working price has been developed for a new agent, if there is potential for it to be brought to the attention of a highly placed critic by a constituent or other individual, the company must investigate ways to avoid the problem or be prepared to address the issue directly with the critic.

These factors and issues will affect every new pricing decision

FIGURE 6. Pricing Considerations for New Pharmaceuticals.

PUBLIC POLICY		
Competition	Disease Characteristics	Value of Therapy
Prescriber Decision Making	PRICE	Patient Characteristics
Company Needs	Reimbursement Environment	Company Abilities
PUBLIC POLICY		

made. Figure 6 provides a summary of these issues in schematic form, with the final price at the center of the chart. Note that the public policy environment surrounds the other considerations. It must be a major consideration in every pharmaceutical pricing decision (19).

REFERENCES

1. Kolassa EM. Physicians' perception of the price and value of frequently prescribed medications. Unpublished.

2. Reekie WD. Pricing new pharmaceutical products. London: Croom Helm, 1977.

3. Brand FN, Smith RT, Brand PA. Effect of economic barriers to medical care on patients' non-compliance. Public Health Rep 1977;92(1):72-8.

4. Shulman NB, Martinez B, Brogan D, Carr AA, Miles CC. Financial cost as an obstacle to hypertension therapy. Am J Public Health 1986;76(9):1105-8.

5. Morisky DE. Nonadherence to medical recommendations for hypertensive patients: problems and potential solutions. J Compliance Health Care 1986;1(1):5-20.

6. Black DM, Brand RJ, Greenlick M, Hughes G, Smith J. Compliance to treatment for hypertension in elderly patients: the SHEP pilot study. J Gerontol 1987;42(5):552-7.

7. Shulman NB, Martinez B, Brogan D, Carr AA, Miles CG. Financial cost as an obstacle to hypertension therapy. Am J Public Health 1986;76:1105-8.

8. Kolassa EM, Smith MC. 1992 National Survey of Hospital Pharmacies: hospital pharmacy directors' ability to use and understand pharmaceutical economic outcomes research. University, MS: Research Institute of Pharmaceutical Sciences, University of Mississippi, March, 1993.

9. Abramowitz PW, Nold EG, Hatfield SM. Use of clinical pharmacists to reduce cefamandole, cefoxitin, and ticarcillin costs. Am J Hosp Pharm 1982;39:1176-80.

10. Hess DA, Mahony CD, Johnson PN, Corrao WM, Fisher AE. Integration of clinical and administrative strategies to reduce expenditures for antimicrobial agents. Am J Hosp Pharm 1990;47:585-91.

11. Miyagawa CI, Rivera JO. Effect of clinical pharmacists' interventions on drug therapy costs in a surgical intensive care unit. Am J Hosp Pharm 1986; 43:3008-13.

12. Chrischilles EA, Helling DK, Aschoff CR. Effect of clinical pharmacy services on the quality of family practice physician prescribing and medication costs. DICP Ann Pharmacother 1989;23:417-21.

13. Lazarus H, Smith MC. After the order is written: pharmacists' interventions in hospital drug therapy. Med Market Media 1988;(May):76-80.

14. Greenfield S, Nelson EC, Zubkoff M, et al. Variations in resource utilization among medical specialties and systems of care: results from the Medical Outcomes Study. JAMA 1992;257:1624-30.

15. Taubman AH, Mason NN. How to price a retail pharmacy's goods and services. In: Tindall W, ed. Retail pharmacy practices. Alexandria, VA: National Association of Retail Druggists, 1989:465-505.

16. Kolassa EM. Physicians' perceptions of drug prices: their accuracy and effect on the prescribing decision. J Res Pharm Econ 1995;6(1):23-37.

17. Holcombe RF, Griffin J. Effects of insurance status on pain medication prescriptions in a hematology/oncology practice. South Med J 1993;86:151-6.

18. Zelnio RN, Gagnon JP. The effects of price information on prescription drug product selection. Drug Intell Clin Pharm 1979;13:156-9.

19. Kolassa EM. The new environment for pharmaceutical pricing. Product Manage Today 1993;(Jan):21-2.

The Role of Price in the Decision to Purchase, Prescribe, or Use Pharmaceuticals

INTRODUCTION

Price elasticity, as a measurable and useful tool for pricing, leaves a lot to be desired, in practical terms. The fact that the price of a product can and will affect sales is unquestionable, but the ability to measure precisely the tradeoff between price and volume must be questioned. The law of demand states: *All things equal, as prices increase, unit sales will decrease, and as prices decrease, unit sales will increase.* The concept behind this law is sound, but not simple. Often overlooked is the qualifying statement: "all things equal." The "things" that are held equal (or constant) are called the determinants of demand, and they define the location and slope of the demand curve. The determinants of demand are:

- Prices of competitive goods or services
- Income or buying power of the customers
- Number of customers
- Customers' tastes and preferences
- Customers' expectations.

These are the "things" that are held constant, and if any of them change, the demand curve also changes. Because these are the factors that determine the demand curve, one must question the

[Haworth co-indexing entry note]: "The Role of Price in the Decision to Purchase, Prescribe, or Use Pharmaceuticals." Kolassa, E. M. (Mick). Co-published simultaneously in *Journal of Pharmaceutical Marketing Practice* (The Pharmaceutical Products Press, an imprint of The Haworth Press, Inc.) Vol. 1, No. 1 (#1), 1997, pp. 63-71; and: *Elements of Pharmaceutical Pricing* (E. M. (Mick) Kolassa) The Pharmaceutical Products Press, an imprint of The Haworth Press, Inc., 1997, pp. 63-71. Single or multiple copies of this article are available for a fee from The Haworth Document Delivery Service [1-800-342-9678, 9:00 a.m. - 5:00 p.m. (EST). E-mail address: getinfo@haworth.com].

likelihood of any of them—much less all—remaining constant for a useful period of time. The ephemeral nature of the demand curve, then, severely limits its practical use.

More important, from a strategic perspective, is that people tend to accept the demand curve as a fixed phenomenon in the market. Studies that purport to measure this curve, even if they could do so with any certainty, simply deliver to decision makers a model that implies they are helpless victims of this curve. These findings compel decision makers to approach the demand curve passively, accepting the implied limits rather than seeking ways to stimulate demand. Consider the typical conjoint study, which simply finds that at a particular price, with a particular set of attributes, your unit sales will be X. You then build your forecasts and marketing plans around this number. You are held hostage by this number. In the quest for precision, we generate numbers that are precisely wrong.

There is little evidence that pharmaceutical markets, generally, are responsive to changes in price levels. Most pharmaceutical markets appear to be extremely inelastic, as the term is understood, in that price reductions, generally, have not resulted in increases in use and price increases have not slowed growth for most products. This does not imply that pharmaceutical markets are not sensitive to price, only that the traditional understanding of elasticity and demand curves has little use in pharmaceutical markets.

The concept of price sensitivity, as opposed to elasticity, is a more qualitative idea—detectable and describable but not measurable to any degree of precision. But by understanding price sensitivity, its variations, and its sources, marketers can manage their markets to overcome or exploit these areas of sensitivity. Understanding price sensitivity allows you to segment the market by differences in sensitivity, to anticipate the effects of sensitivity on your marketing plans and sales success, and to influence the degree and types of sensitivity.

Price sensitivity, in its various forms, has been described by Nagle and Holden, who define ten determinants of price sensitivity:

- Unique value effect
- Perceived substitute effect
- Switching cost effect

- Difficult comparison effect
- Price-quality effect
- Expenditure effect
- Shared cost effect
- End benefit effect
- Fairness effect
- Inventory effect (1).

Each of these ten determinants, or effects, exerts a different influence on decisions to use, prescribe, or purchase pharmaceuticals. Depending on the situation (e.g., patient, payer, product features, etc.), one or more of these determinants will come into play. The marketer can affect the degree to which these effects play a role in decisions or fall victim to them.

Unique Value Effect. The first determinant is called the unique value effect. Buyers (or prescribers or users) are less sensitive to price when they value the unique attributes that differentiate a product from its competitors. For example, Prozac® prescribers (and patients) value the product's "uplifting" effect. Patients with uncomplicated depression are often in need of the uplift the product provides, which is unique among the selective serotonin reuptake inhibitors. Zithromax®, the first once-daily oral broad-spectrum antibiotic, is perceived as very expensive ($7 to $8 per dose), but this dosing delivers such value, in terms of compliance and cure rates, that these features overcome much price sensitivity.

Lescol®'s low price, unique among HMG-CoA reductase inhibitors, is valued by the cash-paying patient; thus, it has a higher share among this group. In this situation, the low price is the product's unique value. Patients with third-party payment plans find this feature of little value. Although pharmacy directors of managed care plans claim to value this feature of Lescol, its lower market share in third-party programs, compared with the cash market, exposes many a pharmacy director's inability to affect product use.

Perceived Substitute Effect. The perceived substitute effect argues that a lack of differentiation among products will increase sensitivity to price when decision makers are aware of the lack of differentiation and of the prices of similar products. Physicians' traditional lack of pricing awareness has acted to prevent this determinant from operating to any great extent in the pharmaceutical marketplace, but those practitioners who are aware of and concerned about costs will act on this information. Firms with me-too products have attempted to make this work for them by pricing their products below prevailing levels and, apparently, hoping the low price would result in use. As Sandoz demonstrated with Lescol, this strategy requires a significant investment in promotion to bring about the necessary level of awareness and interest in the price difference. Firms with relatively undifferentiable products can, as Sandoz has shown, make this effect work for them.

Pharmacoeconomics can play an important role in managing the perceived substitute effect by comparing the costs and effects of a new agent with those of older procedures. When the H_2 inhibitors were first launched, their prices were perceived as high. Then evidence emerged that by reducing the need for surgical repair of ulcers, this class of drugs reduced total health care expenditures significantly. When the cost of the H_2s was compared with the cost of surgery, the drugs appeared downright cheap, and the makers of the H_2s were able to capitalize on the comparison.

This example provides a valuable lesson in the art of properly selecting competition. One must be sure, however, that the costs are truly comparable and that the benefits of reduced costs are seen as such by the decision makers. Saving money by reducing surgeries may not be seen as a benefit by surgeons or by pharmacy directors who may be compensated on the basis of their ability to control spending on drugs.

The perceived substitute effect can also be invoked through direct-to-consumer (DTC) advertising. When Marion Labs (now Hoechst Marion Roussel) launched Cardizem CD® with a direct-to-consumer campaign, they informed patients taking Cardizem SR® of a new option (substitute) that could save them money.

Switching Cost Effect. When users have a "sunk investment" in a product, the switching cost effect is in operation. This is a major reason for the difficulty in moving patients using chronic medications between agents or to generic versions. The efforts in retitration and reestablishing control (or the risk of losing control, in the case of antiepileptics and anticoagulants) act as major deterrents to price appeals. Similarly, a hospital that has made a heavy investment in a specific IV drug delivery system will resist moving to comparable agents that are not available in package configurations compatible with the system in use. The savings to be gained from changing to a new agent are offset by the costs of switching.

Product loyalty brings about switching cost problems for new competitors. A physician who is satisfied with the performance of a particular agent will resist the adoption of a competitive agent for two reasons: the "cost" of learning about the new agent and the "cost" in admitting that the agent they have trusted may not be the best choice. Consumers and other decision makers will act to avoid cognitive dissonance when actions conflict with beliefs (2). They will block out competitive messages to avoid this feeling. Competitors offering new calcium channel blockers (CCBs) found it difficult to dislodge Procardia XL® as market leader because many physicians believed it to be nearly ideal. It took Pfizer, the marketer of Procardia XL, to overtake the product with a new CCB, Norvasc®.

Difficult Comparison Effect. The difficult comparison effect lessens price sensitivity by making straightforward price comparisons difficult. A new class of drugs for treating a condition presently served by another class has the difficult comparison effect in its favor. When Prilosec®, the proton pump inhibitor (PPI) by Astra Merck, entered the market, its mechanism of action–and eventual effectiveness–differed greatly from those of the H_2 inhibitors that dominated the market at that time. Although some early concern was raised about the price of Prilosec, which was significantly higher than those of the H_2s, it was not possible to simply dismiss this new class of drugs because they could not immediately be compared with the older agents.

Similarly, branded products within a chemical class benefit from this effect when a major competitor loses patent protection. Although it is relatively easy to compare branded Tagamet® with generic cimetidine and to make the purchase decision on the basis of the price difference, it is not as straightforward to choose generic cimetidine over branded Zantac®, regardless of the price difference. An examination of the first two years of generic cimetidine competition (Table 1) suggests that, although Zantac's share of H_2 NRx declined slightly (from 54.2% to 51.8%), the prescriptions lost by Zantac went to Pepcid® and Axid®, not to cimetidine. Thus the net

TABLE 1. H_2 Antagonist NRx Activity.

	3q93	4q93	1q94	2q94	3q94	4q94	1q95	2q95	3q95
				Calendar Quarter					
Zantac	54.2%	54.1%	53.9%	52.9%	51.1%	51.6%	51.2%	51.9%	51.8%
Pepcid	14.2%	14.4%	14.6%	14.4%	14.5%	14.9%	15.0%	15.0%	15.6%
Axid	10.5%	10.5%	10.9%	10.6%	10.5%	10.7%	10.8%	10.8%	11.0%
Tagamet	21.1%	21.0%	20.5%	16.4%	6.2%	4.8%	3.9%	3.2%	2.9%
generic cimetidine	0%	0%	0%	5.6%	17.7%	17.9%	19.1%	19.1%	18.8%
total cimetidine	21.1%	21.0%	20.5%	22.0%	23.9%	22.8%	23.0%	22.4%	21.7%

effect of generic cimetidine on Zantac, in the broad outpatient market, has been none. The difficult comparison effect, in a relatively free market, argues against the large-scale loss of sales for a brand when a competitor loses patent protection.

Complicated dosing regimens also induce the difficult comparison effect. Oral agents for the treatment of type II diabetes benefit from difficult comparisons, as the dosing must be individualized. Comparing the price of Precose® and Glucophage® is very difficult simply because the doses for each vary so widely.

Price-Quality Effect. The price-quality effect is a manifestation of the traditional use of price as a surrogate indicator of quality. Lacking other means of quality assessment, consumers often use the price of a product as a measure of its quality. Luxury automobiles are a classic example of this effect. For pharmaceuticals, this effect helps explain the acceptance of the apparently high prices of biotechnology products.

Physicians' general lack of knowledge of the prices of pharmaceuticals may act against this effect as a major force in product use.

In fact, an unpublished study at the University of Mississippi sought to test the hypothesis that physicians use their own assessments of the quality of a product to estimate its price. A study of 200 primary care physicians found a positive correlation (.55) between the physicians' assessment of the quality of a product and their estimates of prices when compared with similar agents.

Expenditure Effect. The expenditure effect argues that the higher the total expenditure of a purchase, the more likely it is that people will seek alternatives. Sandimmune® (cyclosporine, Sandoz) is used to prevent the rejection of transplanted organs. The cost of this product can run between $4,000 and $8,000 per year, depending upon the organ(s) transplanted and the patient's size. Physicians discovered that the use of calcium channel blockers increased the blood levels of Sandimmune, and many sought to use CCBs as a means to reduce the necessary dosing (and cost) of Sandimmune.

On a larger scale, a purchaser such as a hospital buying group, the Veterans Administration, or a large managed care organization will seek first to reduce expenditures that account for a large proportion of its total spending. It is not uncommon for these groups to speak of products coming up on their "radar screen," meaning the expenditures have reached the point where the payers feel obliged to take some action to reduce them. This is the reason antibiotics are a constant focus of cost control in hospitals. It is not that any one agent is so costly but that the total amount spent on antibiotics is so large that payers feel compelled to take some steps to reduce it.

For companies launching new products into markets where the expenditure effect is operative, there are opportunities to exploit the effect by positioning the new product in a way that allows a reduction in total spending. For markets that do not yet show up on the radar screen, marketers need not be unduly concerned that their price will be scrutinized to the point where its sales potential will be severely reduced. This is the reason many orphan drugs are allowed prices that seem inordinately high.

Shared Cost Effect. The shared cost effect is probably the single greatest reason for the paradoxical effect of managed care on the sale of pharmaceuticals. Despite the fears that managed care would restrict access to pharmaceuticals and force prices down, there is ample evidence that managed care has resulted in major increases in the use of higher cost agents. Although this has been discussed elsewhere in this work, it should be stated again that putting a third-party prescription plan into effect reduces patient price sensitivity. The growth of these third-party plans and the subsequent growth of pharmaceutical use are results of the shared cost effect.

End Benefit Effect. The end benefit effect can be divided into two parts: derived demand and the share of total cost. Pharmaceuticals often benefit from the derived demand aspect of the end benefit effect, such as the routine use of broad-spectrum antibiotics in conjunction with surgery or the use of progestational agents to oppose estrogen when the latter is prescribed for menopausal symptoms. Sensitivity to the prices of these agents is less than with many others because their use has become routine as part of the larger therapeutic goal. Related to this aspect of the end benefit effect is the product's share of the total cost of a larger procedure or treatment plan. Among the biggest trends in pharmaceutical markets today is the use of pharmacoeconomics (3). These studies are often used to uncover and promote the net economic or quality of life benefit of the use of a particular agent and to argue that the cost of the agent is inconsequential when related to the total cost of the procedure or when compared with the clinical and economic benefit of the use of the product.

Fairness Effect. The fairness effect is, perhaps, the biggest reason for the criticism of pharmaceutical products in recent years. Buyers will be more sensitive to and critical of prices that are higher than those to which they are accustomed. The initial criticism of the price of Prilosec (discussed earlier) was due in large part to the comparison with the prices of the H_2s, such as Zantac and Tagamet. Similarly, advances in the technology used to derive and purify insulins have brought about significant advances over the older animal insulins. However, the new, short-acting insulins, which more closely mimic the actual performance of native insulin in the patient, have been unable to garner the premiums they should command because of the appearance of fairness: the price of insulin has been established by the older products.

Lacking any other cues, buyers will often use a reference price (not to be confused with the price-control tool used by many governments) to assess the fairness of a price. Pfizer's pricing of Feldene®, the first successful once-daily NSAID for arthritis, brought about outcries of "unfairness," even though the product was priced similarly to other agents, because patients were not accustomed to paying $1 for a single dose. They made the comparison on a pill-for-pill basis and wrongly concluded that Feldene at $1 for a once-daily dose was more costly than Naprosyn®, at $0.50 per dose, taken twice daily.

Inventory Effect. The inventory effect was responsible for the greater part of drug wholesaler profits during the late 1980s. When buyers can store quantities of a product for later use, they are likely to make larger purchases when a low price is available or when they anticipate a price increase. Drug wholesalers learned to anticipate price increases for major pharmaceutical brands and bought heavily prior to the increases. This allowed them to hold the inventory until the price increases and profit significantly from the increases.

CONCLUSION

With an understanding of these aspects and sources of price sensitivity, the pharmaceutical marketer can determine whether there is need for concern about the price of a new agent, or whether there is the potential to use a low price as a positive feature of the product. Some pricing strategies depend upon the presence of one or more of these factors, while others are thwarted because of the marketer's failure to recognize their presence or absence. Rather than simply surrendering to a demand curve, manufacturers should undertake research with users to discover and characterize any price sensitivity effects that may be active in the market and then develop marketing plans that manage these phenomena to the best advantage.

REFERENCES

1. Nagle TT, Holden RK. The strategy and tactics of pricing: a guide to profitable decision making. 2nd ed. Englewood Cliffs, NJ: Prentice-Hall Inc., 1994.

2. Engel JF, Kollat DT, Blackwell RD. Consumer behavior. 3rd ed. Hinsdale, IL: The Dryden Press, 1978.

3. Boston Consulting Group. The changing environment for U.S. pharmaceuticals. New York: Boston Consulting Group, April 1993.

The Pharmaceutical Pricing Research Process

INTRODUCTION

The pricing decision for anything, especially pharmaceutical products, is filled with uncertainty and ambiguity. The price of a medication may have a substantial effect on its adoption and use in the marketplace, but it is equally, if not more, likely to have no effect. It is well established, however, that there are no easy answers, and there is no simple and accurate way of knowing how (or if) the market will respond to the price charged for the product. Pricing research is a logical and necessary approach to reducing–but not eliminating–uncertainty and ambiguity in the pricing decision.

This point is crucial to the understanding of the purpose of pricing research. It will reduce, but not eliminate, uncertainty by providing all the information needed for the decision. No matter how comprehensive the research, a large element of risk remains in the pricing decision.

THE BASIC PROBLEM WITH MOST PHARMACEUTICAL PRICING RESEARCH

The flaws in current pricing research for pharmaceuticals emerge from two sources. First, pricing research tends to be done by mar-

[Haworth co-indexing entry note]: "The Pharmaceutical Pricing Research Process." Kolassa, E. M. (Mick). Co-published simultaneously in *Journal of Pharmaceutical Marketing Practice* (The Pharmaceutical Products Press, an imprint of The Haworth Press, Inc.) Vol. 1, No. 1 (#1), 1997, pp. 73-86; and: *Elements of Pharmaceutical Pricing* (E. M. (Mick) Kolassa) The Pharmaceutical Products Press, an imprint of The Haworth Press, Inc., 1997, pp. 73-86. Single or multiple copies of this article are available for a fee from The Haworth Document Delivery Service [1-800-342-9678, 9:00 a.m. - 5:00 p.m. (EST). E-mail address: getinfo@haworth.com].

keting research professionals, who do not have an in-depth understanding of the dynamics of pharmaceutical pricing issues and thus must simplify the issues to fit their methodologies. Just as important, the research methodologies, in which the researchers place considerable faith, do not accurately reflect the manner in which clinical decisions are reached and tend to overstate the importance of price in the prescribing decision by artificially increasing its visibility to the decision maker.

The final point emerges time and again as the reason for the failure of many products to achieve the sales potential forecasted through pricing research methodologies. When presented with a choice of several prices, any respondent will tend to play the role of the economic person and select the product with the lowest price, other things being equal. The problem arises in that the physician, who is the customary target of such research, tends to have limited pricing information, at best. In practice, the selection of a drug product based on its price conflicts with the fact that the physician often has no idea of the prices of alternatives and with the physician's basic self-image as a healer, which argues against price as a major component of his or her evaluative criteria for product selection. Finally, a single study, regardless of its "comprehensiveness," cannot possibly describe the dynamics of the prescribing decision and the effects of price.

The pricing research process for a pharmaceutical product is, ideally, a series of steps during which a broad range or band of prices is narrowed to a single price or set of prices at which the product will be launched. Despite the desirability of a precise estimate of the price/volume relationship for the product, the decision-making process for the use of pharmaceutical products, globally, precludes the identification of such a function. The precision desired of any study that measures intended use is thwarted by the most basic of the elements of Fishbein's model of behavioral intent, that is, $B \approx BI$ (Behavior is *approximately* equal to *B*ehavioral *I*ntent). That any measure other than that of actual behavior is simply a measure of behavioral intent (which is, by definition, an approximation and not a precise point estimate) precludes the development of a precise model that provides the "optimum" price (1). Instead, the goal of pricing research must be to determine the range of prices within which the unit sales of the product will not be depressed and the firm may profitably sell the product.

In the process of performing studies to determine and narrow this range, a series of questions must be asked. These questions should guide the selection of research methodologies, rather than a procrustean research approach in which the methodology is determined a priori and the question is altered to fit the method, as is too often the case in practice.

Early in the product development process, the first pricing question that must be addressed is: Does there appear to be a relationship between price and product use? Alternatively, the question may be posed as: What role, if any, does price play in product selection? The first step, then, is to address this question.

Secondary data sources, especially commercial audits, are particularly useful at this time, as they allow for the visual and statistical evaluation of the price-market share relationship. The first step is to graph the relationship between price and market share, measured both in total prescriptions and in new prescriptions. The two different prescription measures are necessary because a dominant product in a market may be losing share in new prescriptions while its share of total prescriptions remains high because of ongoing therapy. If such is the case, the price-NRx graph may reflect the difference in prescribing behavior and identify a change in prescriber behavior. Figure 1 provides three potential relationships in hypothetical markets.

FIGURE 1. The Price-Share Relationships in Three Markets.

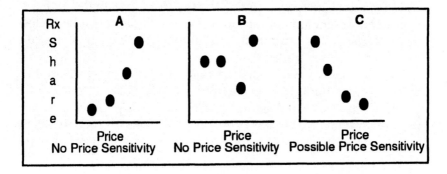

Relationships such as those in Figure 1 would lead to different conclusions. Market A indicates no traditional price-market share relationship, unless one concludes that physicians (or others) select high-priced products over low-priced products because they wish to increase spending. This relationship, incidentally, appears to be the dominant type in most markets–foreign and domestic–and implies that "better" products (those preferred by physicians) are priced according to their value. The graph of Market B indicates no relationship between price and volume. These two markets (A and B) render relationships implying that factors other than price are the major, and perhaps only, determinants of use. Market C displays a relationship that raises the possibility (not certainty) that price plays a major role in product use. In each of these cases, promotional materials of major competitors should be evaluated to determine the positioning used by each, and these should be followed with qualitative research that investigates the role of various prescribing criteria, as well as identification of other entities that affect the prescribing/dispensing decision, such as payer or pharmacy pressure.

A working price range can be established based on this information and the company's own assessment of the likely effectiveness of the product being developed. If the product under consideration will offer substantial improvements over existing (and near-term new) products, appropriate premium prices should be included in the working range.

Realistically, this is all that can be expected in the preclinical/pre-development stage, and the pricing input into the decision at this point must be based on a best guess of the profile of the product and the likely prices of competitive products at the time of launch, which requires the forecasting of competitive prices in the future. A reasonable assumption of a specific price point at this time, unless there is compelling information to argue otherwise, is to use the price of the market leader.

During Phases I and II, pricing (and marketing) research should focus on identifying and evaluating the key decision criteria for product use. This involves developing a list of these criteria and their various levels of intensity and narrowing the list to a workable set of attributes through a process of reduction and ranking (or weighting).

PRODUCT ATTRIBUTES ALONE ARE NOT SUFFICIENT

It should be noted at this point that product attributes alone are not sufficient when forecasting product use, as patient-specific attributes will have at least as great an effect on product choice as the attributes of the product. Physicians will prescribe differently for the elderly, for patients who are known to be noncompliant, or for patients who are unable to afford many medications. Most commonly used survey-based research methods overlook these important attributes in product selection because the "canned" programs often used cannot accommodate this additional level of complexity, which adds a new dimension to the analysis. Still, as this is the way in which products are selected, not posing questions in this manner is to collect data that provide only a portion of the picture. This is the single most compelling argument against the routine use of choice-based trade-off models, such as conjoint and discrete choice, for pricing research.

The recently introduced protease inhibitors for the treatment of AIDS provide an excellent example of the importance of patient attribute over drug attribute. It is well known that these agents, especially when used in combination with other agents, are costly, but it is also known that most patients do not bear the cost themselves. Because of the cost and the limited availability of the products, patient selection is being based on known compliance behavior. The dosing of these products is complex (up to 15 times per day), so patients with a history of poor compliance or whose lifestyles suggest compliance problems will not be started on these agents.

Another example of patient attributes overshadowing product attributes is intervention by managed care plans. It is not uncommon for a physician to prescribe Procardia XL® as the calcium channel blocker of choice, but a patient who belongs to a restrictive managed care plan may be prescribed Adalat CC® simply because that product is reimbursed while the other is not. It is not the attributes of the drug, per se, that drive this decision, but a patient/payer attribute.

Another set of variables often overlooked in pricing research is the dynamic response of the market to changes in marketing efforts.

There is compelling evidence that in relatively nondifferentiated markets, such as H_2 antagonists, ACE inhibitors, and selective serotonin reuptake inhibitors, the availability of samples is *the* key determinant of product selection. Antibiotics, as well, appear sensitive to sample availability and to the recency of sales presentations. Analysis of most markets in which major products have lost patent protection will reveal that the cessation of detailing for the affected brand usually results in a reduction of prescriptions written for the compound that has lost patent protection and a compensating increase in prescriptions for other agents that are still being promoted. Failure to consider these key marketing inputs, arguably the number one source of cost for branded pharmaceutical companies, effectively ignores the impact of the company's programs, and those of its competitors, on the marketplace. It is doubtful that one would wish to argue that it is appropriate to assume, for the sake of forecasting, that these inputs have no effect on product sales. Yet this is exactly what must be assumed when using the choice-based models.

From these observations, one might deduce that a group of dimensions must be modeled to describe the separate effects of patient type, market type, marketing inputs, and product-specific factors (each a separate dimension), and the manners in which product selection is affected by each. These separate models may then be combined to construct a comprehensive model, with the acknowledgment that the errors inherent in each model will combine to create a confidence interval of significant breadth. Figure 2 suggests a way to visualize the drug product selection decision and the effect of the three necessary dimensions.

Identification of these decision criteria and the performance of research to determine the role each may play in the eventual use of the product is the goal at this stage. Logic and experience argue that price will only play a major role in markets in which a number of relatively undifferentiable products compete and in which patients, or some other group, provide significant and consistent price-related feedback to prescribers.

It is important to understand that prescribers, generally, use an evaluative and decision-making process that is sequential in nature (2). Under such a process, called noncompensatory decision mak-

FIGURE 2. The Dimensions of Drug Product Selection for a Market Segment.

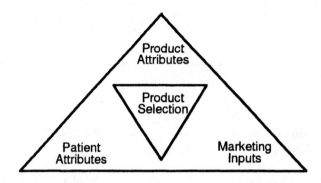

ing, alternative drugs are evaluated on one criterion at a time. All drugs meeting the most important criterion are further evaluated in light of subordinate criteria. Compensatory decision making, on the other hand, involves the simultaneous evaluation of all relevant criteria, a difficult and complex process. It may be argued that under the noncompensatory decision-making process, cost will only be considered when all superordinate criteria are equal for two or more products and that cost will affect the patient.

In a study evaluating the measurement of importance of drug attributes in physician decision making, Chinburapa and colleagues found that when process-tracing techniques, which seek to explain the decision-making process, were compared with conjoint analysis, the measures of attribute importance varied significantly, implying the inability of conjoint measurement to correctly describe the way in which prescribing decisions are made (3). Thus there is evidence that choice-based models are not appropriate when an accurate profile of decision making is required.

Because noncompensatory decision making argues that, in most cases, price will not emerge as a major criterion in the product selection decision, guidance in the pricing decision must come from sources other than the exclusive use of survey-based models. This does not imply that one is free to price the product at several multiples of the prices currently charged, only that within the current range of price there appears to be no price-volume relationship. The question that arises at this point is: How much is too much? This question is based on the assumption of a severely kinked demand curve, as portrayed in Figure 3. When this is the case, the pricing research task is to identify the point of inflection in the curve, the point at which the price begins to harm the sales of the product.

How, then, does one conduct research into this? Because the research problem is to identify and measure the relationship between each of several phenomena and the use of a product, some form of a least squares model, with the proviso that different segments of the market (which could be defined as medical specialty groups, payer types, affiliate nations, or some other delineation) often respond quite differently and may require different models for each segment, could be used. Wind and colleagues, in a study of the diffusion of a new medical technology (CT scanners), concluded that the diffusion of a new health care product varies widely by segment and that aggregate models of the entire market were poor predictors of product performance compared with forecasts made on a segment-by-segment basis (4). Attempts to describe the entire market with a single model are very likely to render unsatisfactory results.

Least squares models and their offshoots, ranging from multiple regression to choice-based models to newer techniques such as neural networks, can prove to be very helpful in price decision making, so long as it is understood that point estimates are only that—estimates. Models that provide some measure of goodness of fit or the proportion of variance explained should be preferred over

FIGURE 3. Proposed Typical Pharmaceutical Product Demand Curve.

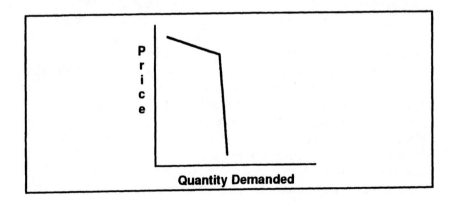

those that do not provide this information. Unfortunately, many of the commercially available choice models do not offer this feature.

In some cases, it may be appropriate to use choice-based trade-off methods such as conjoint or discrete choice models to measure the decision-making process in some segments when the market (patients and payers) is relatively homogeneous and the products are easily differentiable and acknowledged as such by decision makers. Lacking these conditions, choice-based models suffer the shortcomings already mentioned.

When conducting primary research within segments, researchers should consider a multiple regression design before others, as this design allows greater flexibility than many others and the software necessary for the construction and analysis of the regression is readily available from SPSS, SAS, and a number of other sources. When different segments appear to respond differently to the variables tested, a Chow test can be performed among the models of the segments to determine whether they truly require different models or whether an aggregate model may be satisfactory (5). Different prices can be tested within this model by means of monadic testing, in which each respondent is exposed to a single price. In monadic tests, the total sample is divided into subsamples (one for each price tested) to allow testing for differences in responses among the subsamples based on these different price levels.

The presentation of discrete prices in this manner was first suggested by Abrams, who noted response bias problems when respondents were exposed to multiple prices (6). By exposing each respondent to a single price while holding the remainder of the stimuli constant for all respondents, the researcher may test among the groups for differences in purchase intent. Any such differences that emerge can then be attributed solely to the price. This technique has come to be known as a monadic study because of the single price to which each respondent is exposed.

As a general rule of thumb, prices tested should be at least 15% apart. This is based on the observation of the minimum noticeable difference for pharmaceuticals at the retail level (7). A significant difference, where little doubt exists, is in the range of 25% to 35%. This is the reason most generic drugs are launched at prices roughly 30% below that of the brand drug. But even this difference does not guarantee that action will take place in the marketplace because physicians, in general, have shown no interest in prescribing lower cost drugs and pharmacists, or others, often see no advantage in promoting the use of lower cost agents.

In a recent use of the monadic research method with hospital pharmacy directors, where the price of a drug varied from $250 per dose to $3,250 per dose, researchers found that, in this supposedly price-sensitive segment of the market, price did achieve significance as a variable and that variations in product selection were better explained by several other variables (8).

The use of monadic techniques, whether or not they are used in conjunction with multiple regression and other least squares methods, allows the identification of the previously discussed inflection point through a process similar to triangulation. Wide price bands can be tested to determine differences in intent to prescribe (or support or resist prescribing) at the various price points. If no differences in intent emerge among the prices tested, the point of inflection has not been reached. If the highest price tested is at the upper range of prices deemed acceptable to the company, the most likely launch price has been identified. Should the company wish to evaluate the effects of higher prices or to identify the point of inflection, a set of higher prices can be tested.

In a series of proprietary studies, the subjects of which will not be identified, the monadic technique was used to determine the price-volume relationship, or to identify the point of inflection. The products that were the subjects of these studies included neurological agents, respiratory therapies, oncolytics, and immune modulators. In each of these cases, the price-volume relationship either proved to be nonexistent (because the inflection point was not reached) or resembled the demand curve suggested earlier, with the identification of the inflection point.

The same inflection point was identified for the two neurological agents tested (both for chronic, difficult-to-treat disorders). In each case, 4 prices, ranging from $2 to $4 per day, were tested. At prices up to $3 per day (cost to patient), there was no difference in intent to use (or allow the use of) the products. At a daily cost of approximately $3.50 per day, intended use fell dramatically. These products have been launched successfully, but an agent similar to one tested was launched before the test product at a price of $3.75, and its sales have proved disappointing to the company and to Wall Street.

For the respiratory agent, prices between $15.00 and $30.00 (the highest price at which the company would be comfortable) per package were tested. No differences in intended use emerged, and it was concluded that the product could be safely priced at the company's upper limit. A similar finding resulted from the study of the immune modifier.

The study for the oncolytic agent included patient-specific information, which, due to standardization of patients by stage of disease and age, is relatively straightforward and proved to be quite useful. Price resistance emerged for some patient types at some price levels. The study demonstrated that oncologists, globally, would reserve the product for later-stage disease in younger patients at the highest prices and would readily use the product earlier in the disease at lower prices, although slight improvements in efficacy would have significantly enhanced use.

In the case of the oncolytic agent, because population estimates by disease stage were available, a price/volume relationship was attainable. For the other products, where the point of inflection could not be identified or it was concluded that the point had not been reached within the range that was comfortable to the companies, forecasts of sales volume relied on nonprice variables such as promotion, competition, and patient types.

This last point is key to understanding the usefulness of pricing research and the desire to model market potential: the task of pricing research is to determine at which point pricing interrupts the normal process of product diffusion, and other variables will likely be much more important in determining product success.

Because each dimension previously discussed must be profiled differently and pricing may (or may not) play a different role in each, the complexity of the final model may prove daunting. Those wishing to pursue the development of precise comprehensive models would be well served to become acquainted with the concepts underlying chaos theory.

SAMPLE SIZE AND REPRESENTATIVENESS

Any research technique that relies upon samples of the population rather than a census, regardless of quantitative methodologies used, is constrained in its ability to represent accurately the aggregate market by two related factors: size and representativeness. The representativeness of a sample is vital if the results of the research are to be aggregated in an attempt to profile the larger market as a whole. Generally, representativeness is achieved through assurances of randomness, meaning that all members of the population of interest, primary care physicians for example, have an equal likelihood of being included. Any factor that prevents this full participation possibility for all population members violates the assumption of randomness. Because many members of a population of physicians routinely refuse to participate in survey research, the goal of a random sample is impossible to achieve in most medical markets. This violation renders the sample nonrepresentative of the population and devalues the use of the findings as a tool for profiling the aggregate market.

Nonresponders in survey research bring on the risk that this group, whose input is not in the resultant model, may represent a distinct and important segment of the market whose nonparticipation leads to an incomplete picture and an erroneous model. Although the absence of a segment from the sample cannot be totally overcome, the demographic and other categorical attributes of the respondents can be examined for representativeness of the total population, using sources such as *Facts About Family Medicine* or other guides available through medical societies, to weight segments of the respondents to more closely resemble the total market. This weighting partially overcomes the problem of nonrandomness and reduces the level of nonresponse bias, which cannot be accurately measured. This bias increases the error around estimates made from the model and, hence, reduces the precision of the estimate.

Although sample size does affect the representativeness of the sample, the two issues must be addressed separately. Even a purely random sample that is small is likely to provide misleading findings because of sampling error. The optimal sample size for a study to achieve significant findings cannot be known accurately until the data have been collected and analyzed. This is because the estimates are affected not only by the number of respondents but also by the variance in responses to the specific research questions. Responses that vary more broadly require larger sample sizes to achieve statistical confidence and power than questions that elicit very similar responses.

The Central Limit Theorem generally accepts 30 as a minimum sample size (assuming randomness) where average responses will begin to achieve consistency. Larger numbers of respondents reduce the error around the estimates of averages. Should 2 or more groups of 30 respondents each render average responses that are nearly identical, no larger sample sizes are required to conclude that there are no differences between or among the groups. In a monadic study, it is prudent to begin with subsamples of 30 in each group and to perform an interim analysis. Should the responses track very closely, no further research is required. If differences in responses emerge from this initial analysis but, because of the relatively small sample size, the differences do not achieve statistical significance, calculations can be made to determine the minimum necessary sample sizes for the next phase of the research. This calculation is based on the use of the standard error of the mean to measure differences.

The standard error of the mean (*se*) is approximated by dividing the standard deviation of the variable (SD) measured by the square root of the sample size. This figure is then multiplied by 1.96 (the *z*-score for a 95% confidence interval) to determine the presence of significant differences. Thus, if 2 subsamples of 30 each render average estimates of intended use of a new product of 50% and 35% with standard deviations of 25% and 20%, respectively, these differences do not achieve significance:

GROUP	MEAN	SD	*SE*	CONF. INTERVAL
A (*n* = 30)	50%	25%	4.56	41.1% to 58.9%
B (*n* = 30)	35%	20%	3.65	27.8% to 42.2%

Because the confidence intervals overlap, it cannot be concluded that these groups differ in intent to use the product. The mean and standard deviation are relatively stable with a sample of 30 or more, so it is possible to calculate the sample size needed to achieve significance because the standard error is sensitive to sample size.

In this case, increasing each of the subsamples to 50 respondents would render the following:

GROUP	MEAN	SD	*SE*	CONF. INTERVAL
A (*n* = 50)	50%	25%	3.54	43.1% to 56.9%
B (*n* = 50)	35%	20%	2.83	29.5% to 40.5%

The lack of overlap between confidence intervals implies the differences are significant and that the two groups would respond differently. Larger standard deviations would necessitate larger sample sizes to measure such a difference, and smaller standard deviations would require smaller samples. Thus it is possible to begin with a smaller sample to investigate differences and the need to go forward with larger samples. This approach offers the potential to save significant sums of money in the research budget.

This discussion should convince the reader that the generally accepted practice of using a convenience sample of 100 respondents for every study has the potential both to waste money and to generate erroneous models.

REFERENCES

1. Fishbein M. An investigation of the relationships between beliefs about an object and the attitude toward that object. Human Relations 1963;16:233-40.

2. Denig P, Haaijer-Ruskamp FM. Do physicians take cost into account when making prescribing decisions? PharmacoEconomics 1995;8:282-90.

3. Chinburapa V, Larson LN. Assessing drug attribute importance: a comparison of conjoint analysis and process-tracing techniques. J Pharm Market Manage 1993;7(4):3-24.

4. Wind Y, Robertson TS, Fraser C. Industrial product diffusion by market segmentation. Industrial Market Manage 1982;11:1-8.

5. Chow GC. Test of equality between sets of coefficients in two linear equations. Econometrica 1960;28:591-605.

6. Abrams J. A new method for testing pricing decisions. J Marketing Res 1964;28:6-9.

7. Banahan B, Jernigan M. Price sensitivity and generic substitution. University, MS: Research Institute of Pharmaceutical Sciences, University of Mississippi, 1991.

8. Kolassa EM. Hospital pharmacy directors and competing optima: an evaluation of the importance of cost effectiveness versus acquisition price [Dissertation]. University, MS: University of Mississippi, 1995.

The Value of a Pharmaceutical Product

INTRODUCTION

If marketing is defined as identifying and filling the needs of the market, the first important question to ask is: What does the market want? Analysis of the pharmaceutical market in the mid-1990s will show that the market wants:

- Lower costs
- Controllable costs
- Predictable cost
- Improved outcomes.

Note that this list does not include new pharmaceuticals. From the perspective of an institutional buyer–a hospital pharmacist or materials manager or a pharmacy benefit manager–a new drug, in and of itself, is a problem. The effort required to evaluate a new agent and prepare recommendations to adopt or reject it takes time away from other efforts. Often prescribers ignore nonadoption decisions, requiring pharmacists and others to spend more time enforcing formularies and other control mechanisms. For these individuals, then, a new drug means more work.

This is not to say that pharmacists and others are opposed to innovation, but newness in and of itself has no value. The inherent

[Haworth co-indexing entry note]: "The Value of a Pharmaceutical Product." Kolassa, E. M. (Mick). Co-published simultaneously in *Journal of Pharmaceutical Marketing Practice* (The Pharmaceutical Products Press, an imprint of The Haworth Press, Inc.) Vol. 1, No. 1 (#1), 1997, pp. 87-98; and: *Elements of Pharmaceutical Pricing* (E. M. (Mick) Kolassa) The Pharmaceutical Products Press, an imprint of The Haworth Press, Inc., 1997, pp. 87-98. Single or multiple copies of this article are available for a fee from The Haworth Document Delivery Service [1-800-342-9678, 9:00 a.m. - 5:00 p.m. (EST). E-mail address: getinfo@haworth.com].

value of pharmaceuticals is in their efficiency–their ability to render results not available through other methods or at costs significantly lower than those of other interventions. Pharmaceuticals can deliver what the market says it wants, but the lower and/or controllable cost must be documented. This section discusses the link between the economic value of a pharmaceutical agent and the pricing process.

THE VALUE OF A PHARMACEUTICAL PRODUCT

It has been estimated that each year over 600 health economics studies are published and that each pharmaceutical company, on average, begins 23 new studies (1). Although the performance and management of health economic and pharmacoeconomic studies are beyond the scope of this discussion, the basic goal of such studies is to determine the value of pharmaceutical products, and that has much to do with pharmaceutical pricing.

Value-based pricing, which is the most marketing-focused approach to pricing, depends upon accurate valuation of products. But whose value? It is understandable that a company wants to conduct and support research that determines or establishes the maximum value for a product it is about to introduce, but it is important to understand that the value upon which a price should be based is the value to the customer, not the marketer. One must look to a conservative and rather narrow definition of value as a starting point for value-based pricing.

The first, and perhaps most important, price level to determine after the economic studies have been completed is the break-even or zero-based price. This price is derived by modeling the new product into the treatment process, as determined through a burden of illness study, and measuring the difference with and without the new product, which has been assigned a cost of $0. The economic value of the new product is the difference between the two treatment approaches: the cost of the original treatment minus the cost of treatment with the new product. Ideally, the treatment with the new product results in lower costs than treatment without it. The alternative, that treatment with the new product is more costly than treatment without, requires serious decisions about the launch of the product.

At its simplest, the relationship of price to economic value is reflected in the formula:

$$P \leq V$$

where P = price and V = the value of the product. For a purchase to occur, the price charged must be less than or equal to the value perceived by the customer. The lower the price, in relationship to the perceived value, the higher the likelihood of purchase. Several other variables intervene in the purchase decision, of course, but the primary relationship–and concern–is between price and value.

The economic value of the product may have other elements in addition to the basic economic efficiency implied by the break-even level just discussed. Quality differences, in terms of reduced side effects, greater efficacy, or other substantive factors, can result in increases in value beyond the break-even point calculated in a simple cost comparison. Should these factors be present, it is crucial to capture that value in the price of the product. But how much value should be captured? In the pharmaceutical marketing environment of the 1990s and beyond, it is wise to consider surrendering some value to the market–pricing the product at some point below the full economic value of the product. This is appealing for several reasons:

- The measurement of economics is imprecise, and the margin for error can be large.
- If the market is looking for lower costs, filling that need should enhance the market potential of the product.
- From a public relations and public policy perspective, launching a new product with the message that it provides savings to the system can also provide positive press and greater decision-maker awareness.

PRICING AND THE PHARMACOECONOMIC RESEARCH PROCESS

Pharmacoeconomic research efforts should begin early in the product's R&D process, and price-related activities should take place alongside these economic studies. Once a promising compound has been identified, the economic potential of the product should be estimated by first modeling the economic consequences of the disorder. In this way, the economic leverage points in treatment can be identified.

Common economic leverage points are hospital days or visits, physician office visits, and the use of other costly services. If a financial profile of a disorder identifies one or more of these leverage points, the clinical trials of the agent should be aimed at generating reductions in the use of these resources. If your new product can be shown to reduce the need for these services, the economic value and the potential price of your product will be increased.

Once the product has moved into late Phase II and early Phase III testing, the actual effect of the product can be measured or more precisely estimated. Care must be taken to ensure that the economic evaluations are based upon the most likely use and practice for the product, as opposed to protocol-bound use that does not resemble the eventual use in the actual practice setting. The measurement of a distorted value that is driven by a protocol that does not resemble actual practice will lead to incorrect economic findings and a poor pricing decision.

As the likely profile and economic value of the product emerges, some market-based studies of price potential can be undertaken. Qualitatively, focus groups and other methods can be used to gauge price sensitivity or awareness in the market, as well as judging the potential of economic value as a selling point. Should it appear that a high-value appeal has potential as a selling message, various tests can be used to determine the market's acceptance of the product at various prices. The conceptual model for value-based pricing in pharmaceuticals is the simple diagonal graph (Figure 1).

By definition, the currently available treatment (Product A) has a relationship between price (or cost) and effectiveness (or quality) that lies on the diagonal line. A product with lower effectiveness and a higher cost (Product B) would lie to the left of the diagonal line and indicate a product of significantly less value than Product A. Product C has a lower cost and lower effectiveness than Product A, but its value is roughly the same because of its lower price. Product D possesses a lower price and greater effectiveness than

FIGURE 1. Value-Based Pricing Diagonal.

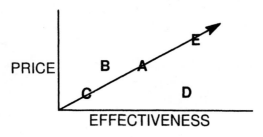

Product A and thus provides the greatest value. If the model is amended as in Figure 2, the conceptual model in the graph allows the user to develop a few pricing scenarios when deciding upon a price.

It must first be acknowledged that values, like prices, are fuzzy–imprecise and not conducive to accurate measurement and reporting. Because of this, the economic value of a product is not a precise figure but a range of values. If Product A, the currently available product, sits on the diagonal, its value lies somewhere in the immediate area around its point on the diagonal. Once the relative effectiveness of a company's product, compared with Product A, has been determined, several potential prices can be tested by comparing their position on the graph with that of Product A. A price that reflects the break-even point will place the product on (or near) the diagonal. In this case, the researcher will have decided to retain all of the economic value of the product and not "share" with the marketplace.

A price that places a product to the left of the diagonal would result in increased costs for the same relative effectiveness. Neither of these scenarios is wrong, per se, because it may be appropriate to charge a higher or equal price. However, it must be acknowledged that such a price/value position can act to slow the adoption of the product into the marketplace and to limit its use.

COORDINATING PRICING AND PHARMACOECONOMICS

Many firms appear to be placing the pricing and pharmacoeconomics functions under common management. Still, in most firms,

FIGURE 2. "Fuzzy" Value.

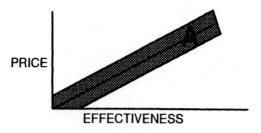

only informal links between the two functions have been established. Those firms with pharmacoeconomics departments residing within the marketing area appear to have more formal relationships between pricing and pharmacoeconomics. The discussion thus far should have pointed out the need for coordination and regular interaction between the two functions. Each needs the other's input, and that need will grow in the future. It is strongly recommended that the consolidation of these two functions under the title of "Market Economics" be considered by every firm.

Three products, in particular, that have entered the market in recent years provide good examples of different value-based approaches, although it is not clear that all three used pharmacoeconomics as the basis for their eventual pricing decisions. Activase® (tPA), from Genentech, entered the market priced at nearly ten times the level of streptokinase, its nearest competitor. This product, which is used solely in the hospital setting, significantly increased the cost of medical treatment of myocardial infarctions, yet the company–and many cardiologists–believed the product to be so valuable, from a clinical perspective, that it would be worth the added cost. The hospitals, which are reimbursed on a capitated basis for the bulk of such procedures, were essentially forced to subsidize the use of the agent, as they were unable to pass the added cost of tPA to many of their patients' insurers. The pricing of the product created a significant controversy, but the sales of Activase have been growing consistently since its launch.

On the other end of the spectrum, Neupogen®, the colony stimulating factor from Amgen, was priced well below its economic value. The product's primary benefit is in the reduction of serious infections in cancer patients, who often suffer large drops in white blood cells due to chemotherapy. By bolstering the white count, Neupogen allows oncologists to use more efficacious doses of cyto- toxic agents while decreasing the rate of infection and subsequent hospitalizations for cancer patients. It has been estimated that Neu- pogen prevents infections that result in an added cost of roughly $6,000 per cancer patient per course of therapy. At roughly $1,400 per course of therapy, Neupogen not only provides better clinical care, but also offers savings of approximately $4,600 per patient.

The economic benefits of the product have helped it to gain acceptance rapidly and with significantly fewer restrictions than products whose economic value is not as readily apparent, such as tPA.

In pricing Imitrex® (sumatriptan), its product for acute migraine headaches, Glaxo reportedly conducted thorough cost of illness studies, measuring the value of workdays lost and other patient- and payer-specific costs. The product is priced in a manner that captures virtually 100% of its economic value. Because patients are very involved in the treatment of migraines (unlike patients who might benefit from the two drugs previously mentioned), the patients per- ceive the value of the product in terms of differences in quality of life and gladly pay any costs not covered by insurers or drug plans.

By contrast, in Europe, the price of sumatriptan has been the object of much criticism from payers. The Danish government, for example, believes its price to be excessive and claims that Glaxo is abusing a dominant position. Some commentators believe that by pricing sumatriptan up to its economic value Glaxo has gone too far. In other words, they believe a lower price would have met less resistance and would have led to earlier reimbursement approval and to more rapid market uptake. Only Glaxo can determine the relative success of its strategy, but sales figures would imply that it is not too disappointed with the performance of the product. In Figure 3, the graph that showed various levels of economic value has been amended below to display the point on the chart occupied by each of the three products just discussed.

Here we have three successful products priced at very different levels relative to their economic value. It should be obvious from

FIGURE 3. Levels of Economic Value.

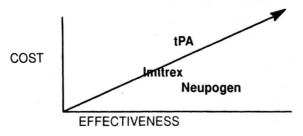

these examples that there is no one best approach to pricing based on economic considerations and that the pricing of each product is unique, with different considerations and different strategies.

It is also important to note that the economic value of an intervention can change. Once a product has been launched into a therapeutic area, the value of that therapy is reestablished based on its presence. The pricing of subsequent market entries affects not only the new products themselves but also the value of previous and succeeding entries. The market for lipid reducers provides clear examples of this.

When Merck launched Mevacor®, the drug was priced well above Questran® (the benchmark product from Bristol-Myers Squibb). At the time, the market for lipid reduction was rather small, and the economics of treating hypercholesterolemia were such that, in pure economic terms, there was no value in treating the disorder. Thus Mevacor was launched at a level that would be considered above the diagonal line on the chart that represents an economic break-even point. But the launch and success of Mevacor reestablished the value of such treatment, providing a new comparator for cost considerations. When Bristol-Myers Squibb launched Pravachol® at approximately the same price as Mevacor, it had priced its agent at the economic break-even point, even though the same price for Mevacor would have been considered a significant premium. Sandoz's launch price for Lescol®, roughly half of Mevacor's, represented a price at or below the economic break-even point, depending upon differences in efficacy. We then have a market that consists of several products with only two prices that have, at times, occupied three different locations on the cost-value chart shown in Figure 4. Value is a moving target, but determining the economic value and break-even point are key steps in reaching appropriate pricing decisions.

Gene Gibson, Associate Director of Pharmacy at the Hospital of the University of Pennsylvania in Philadelphia performs essentially the same analysis as presented above for each new agent. He draws a set of quadrants as shown in Figure 5. As you can see, a new agent that improves outcomes at a lower cost will be accepted immediately, while less effectiveness at a higher cost means instant rejection. The remaining boxes require significant evaluation. Gibson's first question when a new product is introduced: In which box does your product fit?

WHAT IS VALUE?

The preceding discussion of value, like most, tends to address the concept as a fixed and identifiable quantity that is measured, communicated, and accepted by the market. Unfortunately, the concept of value is ambiguous and subjective. The determination of value is subject to many inputs and considerations, and the net value to an individual of a product is affected by several factors. Moreover, what is viewed as valuable to one individual may be seen as a negative product feature to another. Figure 6 presents a conceptual model of the determination of value.

FIGURE 4. Cost/Value for Mevacor, Pravachol, Questran, and Lescol.

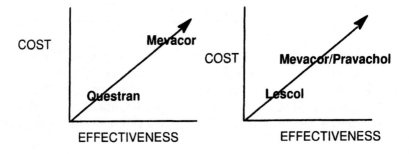

FIGURE 5. Evaluation of a New Agent.

COST

		LOWER	HIGHER
EFFECTIVE-NESS	HIGHER	**ACCEPT**	?
	LOWER	?	**REJECT**

FIGURE 6. The Determination of Value.

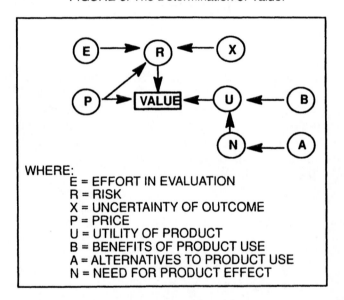

WHERE:
E = EFFORT IN EVALUATION
R = RISK
X = UNCERTAINTY OF OUTCOME
P = PRICE
U = UTILITY OF PRODUCT
B = BENEFITS OF PRODUCT USE
A = ALTERNATIVES TO PRODUCT USE
N = NEED FOR PRODUCT EFFECT

Note first in Figure 6 that the PRICE of the product, heretofore considered to be set according to the value, may actually affect the perceived value. An exceptionally high or low price may, indeed, affect the way a potential buyer assesses the value of the product.

The price also affects the degree of RISK inherent in the purchase. The higher the perceived risk, the lower the perceived value and the less the likelihood that the purchase will take place. The risk is also affected by the EFFORT required to evaluate the product offering. It is generally agreed that decision makers will actively seek to simplify the process of making a decision, and the more effort required to reach that decision, the more negative the decision maker will feel about the object of the decision (2). A value statement that is difficult to interpret and place into the context of the decision maker's frame of reference will increase the effort and risk of the decision and reduce the value of the product.

The degree of risk is also affected by the level of UNCERTAINTY of the final outcome. A value proposition or statement, such as the results of a pharmacoeconomic study, may sound appealing to the marketer, but if the decision maker has doubts that those effects will materialize in actual product use, the value of that information and the value of the product are reduced.

The value of the product is also determined by the UTILITY of the outcome, which in turn is affected by the BENEFITS garnered from that outcome, the NEED for the specific outcome, and the ALTERNATIVES available to reach the same or similar outcome. A product with unique benefits will generally have a higher value than one that competes with several similar products. A product that meets an unsatisfied need, such as the protease inhibitors that reduce the viral load in HIV patients, will be valued more highly than a product that meets a lesser need, such as minoxidil for hair loss. This is not to say that minoxidil is not valuable, only that most will agree that the protease inhibitors meet a much greater need and thus have greater overall value.

Figure 6 represents the process by which a decision maker assesses the value of a product. It is important to remember, however, that for many product purchase and use decisions more than one individual plays a role. The prescribing physician will assess the value of a product in one way, while the payer will use a different set of criteria and value some aspects differently than the prescriber. The patient, in turn, may use completely different criteria to judge the value and benefit of continued compliance. We must understand not only the process of value determination, but also the fact that the various players in the product use decision will each establish value differently.

Identifying the decision makers and their relative influence in the process should be an elementary part of every pharmacoeconomic study and pricing strategy.

REFERENCES

1. Boston Consulting Group. The changing environment for U.S. pharmaceuticals. Boston: Boston Consulting Group, April 1993.

2. Payne JW, Bettman KR, Johnson EJ. The adaptive decision maker. New York: Cambridge University Press, 1993.

Pharmaceutical Pricing
at the Change of Millennia

INTRODUCTION

The pricing of pharmaceuticals, like the pricing of many kinds of products, has traditionally been an uncertain endeavor. Regardless of the information gathered and the research and analysis conducted, one can never be sure that the price decided upon is the correct price. As we approach the millennium, may we expect this specter of uncertainty to remain? Will and Ariel Durant, noted historians of this century, advised: "If you want the present and the future to be different from the past, Spinoza tells us, find out the causes that made it what it was and bring different causes to bear." In business-specific terms, Drucker admonishes: "Long-range planning does not deal with future decisions, but with the future of present decisions." Let us review recent pharmaceutical pricing trends and decisions and consider the extent to which they may affect the future.

THE 1980s

Pricing Decisions

Until very recently, few firms in the pharmaceutical industry committed adequate resources to pricing matters. Although this lack of formal attention to pricing is not unique to the pharmaceuti-

Originally published in *Journal of Pharmaceutical Marketing & Management,* Vol. 1, No. 2/3, 1996. © 1996 by The Haworth Press, Inc. All rights reserved.

[Haworth co-indexing entry note]: "Pharmaceutical Pricing at the Change of Millennia." Kolassa, E. M. (Mick). Co-published simultaneously in *Journal of Pharmaceutical Marketing Practice* (The Pharmaceutical Products Press, an imprint of The Haworth Press, Inc.) Vol. 1, No. 1 (#1), 1997, pp. 99-112; and: *Elements of Pharmaceutical Pricing* (E. M. (Mick) Kolassa) The Pharmaceutical Products Press, an imprint of The Haworth Press, Inc., 1997, pp. 99-112. Single or multiple copies of this article are available for a fee from The Haworth Document Delivery Service [1-800-342-9678, 9:00 a.m. - 5:00 p.m. (EST). E-mail address: getinfo@haworth.com].

cal industry, the lack of a purposeful and coordinated approach to pricing within most firms has, to a great extent, brought about the pricing woes of the present. Pricing has been treated as an event, rather than a process, and each product has been priced in a different way, with pricing research and analysis approaches varying greatly from one product to the next.

Pricing functions and responsibilities were fragmented within most firms, with product managers and/or marketing research departments responsible for the bulk of analysis and consideration and top managers, relying on instinct, setting the list price for launch. Once commercialized, the price of the products tended to go in two directions, with list prices increasing at a fairly regular rate and contract prices, often managed by sales functions, continually moving downward in response to pressures (both real and imagined) in growing price-sensitive market segments.

These pricing activities tended to be performed in a discrete manner, with little or no coordination among the various parties and precious little coordination between the pricing strategy and the marketing plan for the products. Thus, it was not uncommon for marketing campaigns to tout a product's unique benefits and clinical value and point out the lack of appropriate alternatives while selling functions were busily discounting the same product to hospitals, nursing homes, and managed care groups, choosing to compete on price with older–even generic–agents.

These and other phenomena have interacted over the past 15 years to bring about the pricing environment currently faced by pharmaceutical makers. The use of generic drugs began to grow as a force in the early 1980s, and manufacturers of branded pharmaceuticals soon discovered that they could substantially raise the prices of their off-patent products without suffering severe losses in unit sales, beyond those already lost to generics, and thereby preserve sales levels as unit sales declined (1). This lack of price elasticity was due to two circumstances: the generally low prices for pharmaceuticals at the time and the traditional lack of price sensitivity by prescribing physicians (2). Manufacturers soon began to increase prices for patent protected products at nearly the same rate used for multisource drugs and, again, suffered no ill consequences, commercially. Simultaneously, they began to price new products at significant premiums over existing agents (3).

This rate of price growth, however, was noted by several public officials, including Senator David Pryor of Arkansas (4). Government hearings and investigations, together with attention by the media, brought great pressure on the American drug industry to change its pricing behavior.

It has long been accepted that new pharmaceutical products will enter the market at prices higher than those products preceding them to the market (5, 6). That both the pharmaceutical industry's chief critic, Senator Pryor, and the editor of the trade magazine serving the executives of that industry held the same conception of initial product pricing bears this out (7). Senator Pryor, in a 1990 *Health Affairs* article entitled "A Prescription for Higher Drug Prices," stated: "Rarely is a new product priced at a significantly lower level to attract market share from its competitors." John Curran, editor of *Pharmaceutical Executive*, noted the "new" pricing approach taken by Merck in the launch of Vasotec®, which was priced below its competitor, unlike other new agents (7). There appears to be a basic assumption among casual observers and critics alike that new agents will be priced higher than the older agents they are intended to replace in the market. But this trend has reversed itself.

A study by the Boston Consulting Group found that 21 of the 24 new chemical entities with direct competition that were introduced in the United States in 1991 and 1992 were priced, on average, 14% below the leading product in their class (8). For the most active chronic therapeutic areas, which include antihypertensives and other cardiovascular products, the discount averaged 36%. An investigation by researchers at the University of Mississippi found that only one product has been priced at a premium to direct competition since 1992 (3). This is a marked departure from the traditional and assumed pricing behavior of the past.

This change also leads us to challenge a general assumption about pharmaceutical prices—that generic products are less costly than brands. Grabowski and Vernon found that the prices for chemically equivalent generic versions of branded products varied in price by up to 50%, a finding that, according to economic theory, is not expected in a "commodity market" (9). Bloom and colleagues found that generic versions of branded pharmaceutical products were not always priced below the brand (10). In 66% of the products studied, the highest retail price found for generics was above the lowest price found for the brand of the same chemical makeup. While this study was based on a multipharmacy sample and there were no individual stores in which the price of the generic was higher than that of the competing brand, the distribution of retail prices was such that it could be concluded that generics are not always less costly than their branded counterparts.

Given that manufacturers have begun to set the prices of some of their newer products well below those of established brands and that it is the older, established brands that will receive generic competition because their patents will usually expire before those of their newer competitors, it is not unlikely that some new brands would be less costly than generic versions of some older competing products. This statement would seem to defy what might be considered common wisdom, but it can be demonstrated that some newer brands are, indeed, less costly than generic versions of their older competitors. A review of the National Prescription Audit and the pharmaceutical pricing database Price Check-PC reveals that the generic versions of nifedipine and diltiazem, two popular calcium channel blockers, at $1.17 and $1.47 per day, respectively, are priced above the newer branded calcium channel blockers Dyna-Circ® (isradipine, Sandoz, $1.04/day), Plendil® (felodipine, Astra-Merck, $0.92/day), and even an older brand, Calan SR® (verapamil, Searle, $1.16/day) (11, 12).

Even as the prices of newer agents have moderated the rate of price growth, the emergence of managed health care and hospital buying groups has brought about significant changes in the way in which pharmaceutical prices are determined. Aggressive bidding has caused a wide disparity between the retail prices and special contract prices of many pharmaceuticals (13). It appears to have become routine to offer discounts to specific customers.

The imposition of mandatory rebates based on discounts offered to other customers and paid to Medicaid programs, however, appears to have caused many firms to rethink their discount policies, as many have begun to increase prices to these segments (14, 15).

Newly emerged pressure in the form of pharmacy and legislative accusations of discriminatory pricing has resulted in calls for "unitary pricing" to further narrow the discount gap.

Perhaps the most profound change in the pharmaceutical pricing environment in the 1980s was that the prescriber's choice of drug therapy came under the influence of payers and other intermediaries (16). Managed care, as opposed to traditional fee-for-service health insurance, grew from covering 5% of the insured population in the United States in 1980 to 80% of the insured population in 1991 (8). The growth of cost consciousness among payers appears to be a major force behind the change in the way manufacturers are setting their initial prices.

Finally, the useful life of pharmaceutical products has declined rapidly over the past 15 years. Early generic erosion and more direct competitors have brought about a shortened commercial life for a product, and lengthier times for approval have delayed the entry of many new products. As a result, the average pharmaceutical product has a "useful" life of approximately seven years (9). It is during this period of useful life that the product must generate sales and profits sufficient to finance the discovery and development of newer agents. Such a situation would appear to require higher than traditional prices if newer products are to be discovered.

Thus, the most recent trends in pharmaceutical pricing seem to be the combination of the moderation of price growth and the narrowing of discount ranges with increased need for price flexibility.

The Expansion of Price Controls

Concurrent with the rise and fall of price growth in the United States, health care systems in other nations began to assert significant and growing control over pharmaceutical prices. Nations in northern Europe such as Germany, the Netherlands, and many Scandinavian nations, which began the decade of the 1980s with relatively free pricing for pharmaceuticals, began the decade of the 1990s with increasing restrictions (17). Contrasted with price growth in the U.S., which far exceeded the general rate of inflation during the 1980s, real prices for pharmaceuticals fell, relative to other goods and services, in most European nations (1). Even with this result–deflation of pharmaceutical prices–every European government has tightened controls over pharmaceutical prices in recent years.

It appears that government officials often confuse total spending with pricing problems, assuming that spending growth indicates excessive prices. Evaluation of European price control systems by the U.S. General Accounting Office has concluded that these programs are insufficient to control drug spending because, despite holding price growth below prevailing rates of inflation, total spending on pharmaceuticals continued to increase faster than the rate desired (18). Although such evaluations appear to ignore the inherent cost-effectiveness of pharmaceuticals and fail to consider the cost and quality consequences of the underutilization of prescription medications, these issues do not seem to affect decision making within government bodies (19).

A regulatory approach common to many nations is "reference pricing." Under such a system, the prices charged for a pharmaceutical product in several different nations are compared by a regulatory agency to assure that the prices charged in that nation are roughly equivalent to those charged in other nations. Canada, Portugal, and Italy now use such a system, and it appears likely that reference pricing will be adopted in the near future by Germany, the United Kingdom, and other nations.

The range of prices charged for the same product in different nations has been studied exhaustively, and it is often found that drug prices in the United States are higher than elsewhere (20, 21). Comparisons of international drug prices, often commissioned by the federal government, have brought about calls for a reference pricing system in the U.S (21). A reference pricing system was prominently featured in the Clinton Health Plan of 1994. Although no such system is now in place, large disparities between prices in the U.S. and other nations will continue to be brought to the attention of regulators. A narrowing of international price "bands" appears to be in the works.

Many publicly financed health care provision systems were developed as government responses to the perceived problem of unmet medical need (22). While public officials in the United States often note the growth of Medicaid spending, especially for pharmaceuticals, and point to this growth as an indication of the need for tighter controls on health care costs, few have acknowledged the inevitability of cost increases in a system that provides goods and services free of charge (5, 23). As a former Minister of the British National Health Service noted, "There is virtually no limit to the amount of free medical care an individual is capable of absorbing."

Although the many programs provide a comprehensive package of health care goods and services and are meant to provide an overall benefit, the components of the benefit are often budgeted and managed as separate entities, resulting in conflicts between budgetary authorities (24). Many private insurers providing a pharmaceutical benefit operate the pharmacy program as a "carve out." This means that the pharmaceutical benefit is managed separately from the other aspects of the system. Thus, it has become common that the greater good of the total system is often subordinate to individual budget performance.

The budgetary problems of many government-provided health care programs are manifestations of a basic paradox in public transfer payment systems: as economic output and available tax revenues decrease, the demand for government assistance increases (22). Hence, as the demand for medical benefits–including pharmaceuticals–increases, the funds available to support those benefits are decreasing (25). Budgetary "crisis" in such a system is virtually guaranteed.

Over the past decade, studies have demonstrated that tight budgetary control of pharmaceuticals often results in increases in spending on other health care goods and services to offset any savings on drugs, a phenomenon known as the service substitution effect (26, 27). Other studies by Moore and Newman and Smith and Simmons have shown that the imposition of these controls does not even guarantee a reduction in spending on pharmaceuticals (28, 29). While some other studies in this area were questioned for their assumptions or methodologies, few studies have been produced that establish the ability of a restrictive formulary alone to save money in an outpatient setting (30).

Several cost control schemes, such as monthly prescription limitations and cost sharing, have also been shown to be less than optimal in controlling costs. As Nelson, Reeder, and Dickson found, restrictions or cost sharing can result in problems of underutilization, and underutilization can have a negative effect on health and result in cost increases (31). The imposition of a maximum number of prescriptions per beneficiary has been shown to have severe negative consequences, increasing total costs by increasing hospitalizations and nursing home admissions (32). Despite the preponderance of evidence that such restrictions are counterproductive, both in financial and health status terms, the bureaucratic faith in budgetary fragmentation appears unlikely to be shaken, and the continued micromanagement of the prescription budget can be expected in the future.

Thus, the key decision makers in prescription drug use appear to treat price in conflicting ways: physicians, in general, pay no attention to the price of a product, while other intermediaries can be said to consider little else. Price, then, plays very different roles in decision making, and firms must balance these opposing forces when setting prices.

Pharmacoeconomics

In response to pricing pressures and to provide more information about their products, most pharmaceutical firms operating in the United States are, to some extent, engaged in pharmacoeconomic research. Although the field of pharmacoeconomic research is still in its relative infancy, there appears to be great hope that such studies will provide an appropriate basis for judging the economic value of pharmaceutical agents, as well as other health care interventions.

THE FUTURE

The future environment that faces pharmaceutical manufacturers will be determined by the actions of customers, regulators, and the firms themselves. To expect significant changes in the decision-making and evaluative process of the governments is, perhaps, naive. It is thus incumbent upon the pharmaceutical firms and others to adapt to the decision-making styles of these officials.

The current trends that, if left unchallenged, are likely to continue include:

- Narrowing of the range of prices charged in different nations
- Further consolidation of buyers into more powerful groups
- More nonphysician decision makers
- Continued growth of generic drugs
- Continued increases in health care spending and scrutiny of drug budgets
- More attempts by pharmaceutical manufacturers to use price as a selling point
- Continued demands for discounts by many customers.

These combined–and often contradictory–trends will shape the pricing environment of the future. Many of the trends, several of which are troublesome for pharmaceutical makers, are self-imposed. Left unchecked or unchallenged, they will lead to a general lowering of price levels in the United States.

A seemingly ideal pricing environment would be one in which the value of pharmaceuticals is acknowledged and accepted and the prices are set according to the value of the product. Such an environment would clarify the "rules" for price determination and allow customers to evaluate the adoption of a new product. Pharmacoeconomic studies can facilitate such an environment if those sponsoring and performing such studies can agree on meaningful endpoints and health care administrators will admit that reductions in the pharmacy budget do not necessarily result in lower costs overall. The establishment of the economic value of a new pharmaceutical product would allow for a rational, transparent mechanism for the pricing decision, and we must continue to work for the acceptance of these studies. But three major factors, each emanating from regulatory bodies, stand in the way of value-based, rational pricing of pharmaceuticals. The first two factors are associated with price differentials among nations.

International price disparities will remain an issue of contention between those producing pharmaceuticals and those purchasing them. There are two distinct areas of concern: price differentials among developed nations and differences between the prices charged in developed versus undeveloped nations. The range of prices charged for the same medication in Europe can be quite broad. It is not uncommon that prices in France, Spain, and Greece are less than half the prices charged in Germany, the Scandinavian countries, or the United Kingdom. Such disparities will not be tolerated for long; thus, it is imperative that the price levels of pharmaceuticals in southern Europe be brought up to approach those in northern Europe and the United States. Failure to address this disparity will eventually lead to a downward adjustment of prices in the nations of northern Europe and North America.

As we look to emerging markets, on the other hand, price disparities will become a necessity. Regardless of the outcome of "price harmonization" in Europe, it must be admitted by producers and national authorities that citizens and governments of emerging nations cannot afford to pay the full value for many medical technologies. Part of the reason for this is that the current lack of health care technology in many nations implies the relatively low value, in economic terms, of health care interventions in general. Access to modern medicine, however, can help to free resources and to provide economic stimulation. But this cannot occur if emerging nations cannot afford to pay prices that are affordable in developed nations. For example, treatment for a disorder such as hepatitis is costly in developed nations, and a hepatitis cure could well be worth $1,000 or more per patient. But nations such as China, where the incidence of hepatitis is much greater than in the U.S. or Europe, may not be able to afford the $1,000 per patient because (1) that is far beyond what they now spend to treat the disorder and (2) national priorities are such that the funds that would be required to treat all appropriate patients could better be spent in other areas. In such cases, authorities in the developed countries must allow the product to be sold at its economic value ($1,000+) in their nations while it is being sold at a significantly lower price in China. Demands for price equity among all nations will deny needed medication to some nations and/or prevent drug manufacturers from earning the profits necessary to fuel the discovery and development of new agents.

The need to earn profits to fuel new drug discovery brings us to the last of the three factors: patent life. As periods of regulatory review and the time needed to comply with new government-imposed research requirements have lengthened, the effective patent life of a drug in the United States has become dangerously short.

The trends toward lower prices at product launch and slower price growth, when combined with shortened periods of exclusivity, bring about the real danger that few new drugs will ever generate revenues sufficient to fund ongoing R&D. Clearly, new R&D efficiencies and/or initiatives that lengthen the period of exclusivity are necessary if drug discovery and development is to continue and research-based companies are to survive. A single year of extended exclusivity is worth approximately 18% of the average product's sales, or price. Each additional year of exclusivity, on average, generates as much profit as an average selling price that is 18% higher. Clearly, lower launch prices demand longer exclusivity.

The Value of Pharmaceuticals

The main impediment to the appropriate and equitable pricing of pharmaceuticals lies in society's lack of acknowledgment of the value of pharmaceuticals, both in the macro sense–the financial savings gained through the use of pharmaceutical products as a whole–and from a micro perspective–the financial and patient-specific benefits from the appropriate use of many, if not most, new drugs. Part of the problem lies in the failure of society to take a systemwide view when evaluating health care, part in the long-term demonization of the pharmaceutical industry by critics, and a great deal in the industry itself.

The first two issues are self-explanatory; the third, and by far the most damaging, issue requires some discussion. Most pharmaceutical companies have actively worked in ways that devalue pharmaceutical products. The companies' own conduct has reduced the value of medications in the eyes of customers and society at large. For the past several years, prices in pharmaceutical markets have gone in two directions: increasing or holding firm in outpatient, cash-based markets and charging lower prices in hospital and managed care markets. Although these lower prices are in response to perceived market demands and are often accompanied by well-reasoned strategies for the discounts, public knowledge of these multi-tiered prices has brought many to question the appropriateness and equity of the nondiscounted prices. Regardless of the legality of multiple price levels, which has been upheld time and again, two observations must be made:

1. There is little evidence that the deep discounting associated with managed care contracts has substantially affected the use of pharmaceutical products. In most therapeutic areas, the market share for individual products is the same in managed care markets as in cash markets.
2. The act of discounting, especially at some of the levels reported, signals (rightly or wrongly) that the company is willing to accept less for its product than it charges those who do not benefit from discounts. This is interpreted as over-charging.

Pharmaceutical firms must consider the financial and political consequences of pricing decisions and recognize that the granting of discounts is a pricing decision that cannot be made without careful consideration of the effect of those discounts on all aspects of the business. Firms must work to rationalize and manage all pricing activities while simultaneously working with public officials to recognize the value of pharmaceuticals as a cost control tool. I am afraid, however, that this value will not be acknowledged as long as perceptions of unfair pricing, brought on by wide price ranges, continue to exist.

REFERENCES

1. Grabowski H, Vernon J. A sensitivity analysis of expected profitability of pharmaceutical research and development. Manage Dec Econ 1992;3(1):36-40.
2. Zelnio RN, Gagnon JP. The effects of price information on prescription drug product selection. Drug Intell Clin Pharm 1979;13:156-9.
3. Chukkapalli R, Kolassa EM, Ogilvey S, Hayman-Taylor T. The 15 year trend in prices at launch for outpatient prescription medications. Unpublished.
4. U.S. Senate. Special Committee on Aging. Prescription drug prices: are we getting our money's worth? Serial No. 101-F. Washington, DC, 1992.
5. Pryor D. A prescription for high drug prices. Health Aff 1990;9:101-9.
6. Dranove D. Medicaid drug formulary restrictions. J Law Econ 1989; 23:143-62.
7. Curran JP. Strategic shifts in pricing policies. Pharm Exec 1986;6(Apr):92-4.
8. Boston Consulting Group. The changing environment for U.S. pharmaceuticals. New York: Boston Consulting Group, April 1993.
9. Grabowski HG, Vernon JM. Brand loyalty, entry, and price competition in pharmaceuticals after the 1984 Drug Act. J Law Econ 1992;23:331-50.
10. Bloom BS, Wierz DJ, Pauly MV. Cost and price of comparable branded and generic pharmaceuticals. JAMA 1986;256:2523-30.

11. IMS America. National Prescription Audit. October-December 1994. Plymouth Meeting, PA: IMS America.

12. Medispan Inc. Price Check-PC. December 1994. Indianapolis, IN: Medispan Inc.

13. Pathak DS, Klinger PA. Predictive factors in bid purchasing of antibiotics. Top Hosp Pharm Manage 1981;1(1):17-28.

14. Taylor S, Kucukarslan S, Sherrin T. Evidence and response to the impact of the Medicaid Drug Rebate Program (OBRA) on hospital pharmacy: a progress report from central Ohio. Hosp Pharm 1991;26:621-5.

15. Palumbo FB, Schondelmeyer SW, Miller DW, Speedie SM. Battered bottom lines: the impact of eroding pharmaceutical discounts on health-care institutions. Am J Hosp Pharm 1992;49:1177-85.

16. Wilensky GR, Blumberg LJ, Neumann PJ. Chapter 4. Pharmaceuticals and decision-making in the United States: cost consciousness and the changing locus of control. In: van Eimeren W, Horisberger B, eds. Socioeconomic evaluation of drug therapy. Berlin, New York: Springer-Verlag,1988:32-45.

17. Wertheimer AI, Grumer SK. Overview of international pharmacy pricing. PharmacoEconomics 1992;2:449-55.

18. Anon. European price controls not sufficient to control drug spending without policies in place to control use. FDC Rep–Pinksheet 1994;(Jul 4):7-9.

19. Brown RE, Luce BR. The value of pharmaceuticals: a study of selected conditions to measure the contribution of pharmaceuticals to health status. Washington, DC: Battelle Medical Technology and Policy Research Center, March 1990.

20. Andersson F, McMenamin P. International price comparisons of pharmaceuticals–a review of methodological issues. London and Washington, DC: Battelle Medical Technology and Policy Centre (MEDTAP), 1992.

21. U.S. General Accounting Office. Prescription drugs: companies typically charge more in the United States than in Canada. Report to the Chairman, House Subcommittee on Health and the Environment, Committee on Energy and Commerce. GAO/HRD-920119. Washington, DC: September 1992.

22. Soumerai SB, Ross-Degnan D. Experience of state drug benefit programs. Health Aff 1990;9:36-54.

23. Goodman JC, Dolan EG. Economics of public policy. St. Paul, MN: West Publishing Company, 1985.

24. Kozma CM, Reeder CE, Lingle EW. Expanding Medicaid drug formulary coverage: effects on utilization of related services. Med Care 1990;28:963-76.

25. Reutzel TJ. The nature and consequences of policies intended to contain costs in outpatient drug insurance programs. Clin Ther 1993;15:752-64.

26. Bloom BS, Jacobs J. Cost effects of restricting cost-effective therapy. Med Care 1985;23:872-80.

27. Hefner DL. Cost effectiveness of a restrictive drug formulary. Washington, DC: National Pharmaceutical Council, 1980.

28. Moore WJ, Newman RJ. U.S. Medicaid drug formularies: do they work? PharmacoEconomics 1992;1(Suppl 1):28-31.

29. Smith MC, Simmons S. A study of the effects of formulary limitations in Medicaid programs. Admin Policy J 1982;2:169-98.

30. Rucker TD, Morse ML. The Medicaid drug program in Louisiana: critique of the Hefner-Pracon Study. Am J Hosp Pharm 1980;37:1350-3.

31. Nelson AA, Reeder CE, Dickson WM. The effect of a Medicaid drug copayment program on the utilization of prescription services. Med Care 1984;22:724-36.

32. Soumerai SB, Avorn J, Ross-Degnan D, Gortmaker S. Payment restrictions for prescription drugs under Medicaid: effects on therapy, cost, and equity. N Engl J Med 1987;317:550-6.

Index